Omega 3 and vitamin D secrets!

Omega 3 and vitamin D secrets!

How do you obtain a healthy level of Omega 3 and vitamin D these days?

Svein Torgersbraten

authorHOUSE®

AuthorHouse™
1663 Liberty Drive
Bloomington, IN 47403
www.authorhouse.com
Phone: 1-800-839-8640

First published by AuthorHouse   07/18/2011

ISBN: 978-1-4567-8198-9 (sc)
ISBN: 978-1-4567-8199-6 (ebk)

Printed in the United States of America

This book is printed on acid-free paper.

Contents

Background

The information on how to obtain a healthy level of Omega 3 and vitamin D to eliminate dry skin and body was discovered by one doctor in biochemistry in the USA during the 1940s in his search to find natural cures for illnesses caused by the lack of the lipids Omega 3 and the oil soluble vitamin A and D.

For whatever reason, his important discovery and solution to obtain a healthy level of the essential fatty acid Omega 3 and the oil soluble vitamin A and D from food and supplements has remained a secret to most people.

Since the discovery of the oil soluble vitamins and the essential fatty acids in the early years of 1900 it has been known the cells in our skin and body need Omega 3 and vitamin D and the other oil soluble vitamins to stay healthy. There is however no information on how to obtain a healthy level of these important lipids, except the old recommendations to eat food or take supplements rich in these lipids. If we follow this old recommendation we still get dry skin and body and illnesses related to the lack of these important lipids.

I became aware of his discovery by chance recently, during my ongoing study of cancer which started back in early 1995, when my first wife, Margaret, was diagnosed with cancer. At that time I promised myself to study cancer and health until I reach an understanding of cancer. With my study of cancer I discover health information, which might not be directly related to cancer, which I think is essential for good health. This book contains such information. Should you have dry skin and body or be interested to obtain a healthy level of Omega 3 and vitamin D to protect your health and you take the time to read the book and the time to test it out I think you will agree with me. This information is essential for good health.

I guess most of us when we reach a certain age feel that we have something inside us which we know is not as it should be, even if we feel healthy. We accept it as one of these irritants or issues which can not be eliminated with the many modern pills, creams or medicines available, as it always come back, whatever we try or do.

In this respect I would like to refer to an advertisement in the "Financial Times"/ UK in May 1997 by Hoechst. Hoechst was one of the largest pharmaceutical companies in Germany at the time, where they informed 2/3 of all illnesses are incurable. What a surprise, I thought. That means only 1/3 of all illnesses do have a medical cure. I guess this is why we are having health issues without a medical solution based on pharmaceutical medicine.

Some of these health issues are new and some have probably existed for hundreds of years or perhaps even much longer. Some of them most likely had simple natural healing solutions discovered by chance or research by doctors or other health related people at the time. In our modern society with a relative new pharmaceutical industry focusing their production of medicine on chemical products, which are known to have various side effects, most of these natural healing methods or medicines have unfortunately been forgotten by most doctors and people.

The internet is changing this, so there is still a good chance that many of the unsolved illnesses can be solved with a simple natural cure one day, with the help of some old health documents, copied and uploaded on the internet.

Svein Torgersbraten

2

Disclaimer

I am not a health professional, but an engineer with a B.Sc. degree in Electrical Engineering from a university in Scotland/UK. I have worked in engineering, marketing and corporate management for large international companies in different countries most of my life.

My only background in health is my ongoing study of cancer which started back in 1995 when my first wife Margaret was diagnosed with cancer. The aim with my study is to reach an understanding of cancer and health. With my study I discover sometimes information which I consider very important for health. With the right understanding I think the information in this document could benefit the health for a lot of people. For this reason I decided to make it available for information and education. This document should not be considered as a medical document or medical advice by anyone. In case you have questions about your health please consult a health professional.

Hopefully the document will give you some new information and ideas on how you can improve your health the natural way. It is however important to understand that if you start something new you must take into account your own actual health condition as it seems that our bodies are all mostly the same, but different. In other words, what worked for me might not work for you, and what worked for someone else may not work for you either without some added effort from your side, so consider the following message, which I have copied, from a man in Japan who faced the most difficult illnesses including cancer and survived:

"Health is not a gift, but something each person is responsible for through his or her own daily effort"
-Ryuseki Nakayama, chlorella-therapy.com

Svein Torgersbraten
www.omega3andvitamindsecrets.com

Lack of lipids in the cell membranes cause dry skin and body and associated illnesses.

Your skin is the largest organ in your body and through its different skin layers the skin performs different functions and helps to regulate your body temperature. The skin layers contain billions of cells, millions of sweat glands, hair follicle, sebaceous glands, nerve endings and blood vessels.

The cells in your skin, like the trillions of cells in the rest of your body, depend on proper nutrients to function properly. Without proper nutrients, the cells will over time start to starve, dry out and malfunction.

The cell membranes need water and what is defined as essential fatty acid Omega 3 and the oil soluble vitamin A and D and other lipids and nutrients. You discover it normally first by dry and flaky skin on hands, face, legs and hard skin on the heel of your feet and then gradually the skin in your face start to dry out and wrinkle.

We start to apply various lotions or oils to the outside of the skin to try to correct the drying out process of the skin, but we know it work only temporarily, as we have to repeat it regularly.

The drying out of the skin or the cell membranes in the cells of the skin is the dryness we see, but the dryness is much more than skin deep as the lack of the correct lipids affects every cell in the body.

In this respect doctors used to say that your skin is the barometer of your health, as it mirrors the condition of your whole body. Dry skin for them was a sure sign of a dry body or dry cells in the body.

The lack of lubrication or lipids in the cells and their cell membranes can over time cause much more harm than the dry skin and the few wrinkles we see.

The list of illnesses which doctors these days relate to the lack of the essential fatty acid Omega 3 with its DHA and EPA and the oil soluble vitamin D is getting longer each year. Ongoing medical research of illnesses and new understanding of the influence of Omega 3 and vitamin D on health add to the list. To get a brief overview of the most common illness due to lack of these important nutrients a list of illnesses is included in one of the next chapters. Illnesses related to lack of the oil soluble vitamin A seems to be rare with our current diet and is not included.

So what do we normally do to obtain the lipids Omega 3 and vitamin D?

We try perhaps to eat fish each week as we know fat fish is a good source of these lipids, but rarely do we see or feel any difference in our skin after eating the fish. These days the increased fish eating can be even more difficult to accept for some people with the news full of information about eating less fish due to the widespread mercury contamination of the sea and the fish. To avoid the mercury contamination in the fish we might also try to eat more of the fat and pink salmon supplied from one of the many fish farms, hoping that it would have less mercury and be better than the wild fish, but still we do not see or feel a difference in our skin. The same happens when we eat other food also rich in these lipids. Still no difference.

We might also try to spend more time in the sun, to produce vitamin D in our skin, but we might be too worried by all the information produced by various interest groups recommending us to use sun blocking cream or lotion so we follow this advice. In the end we might not get much benefit from this natural and healthy source of vitamin D.

In desperation or perhaps because of childhood memories of being forced to take Cod liver oil or fish oil, we start perhaps to take this type of marine oil, preferably in capsule form to avoid the strange flavour, and even in the liquid form, but again we do not really see or feel a difference in our dry skin or body.

How do you eliminate dry skin or the dry cell membranes in the cells of the skin?

But more important is probably the following which you might not even have thought about yet: How do you eliminate the dry conditions of the other cell membranes in the trillions of cells below your skin?

Doctors in the early years of 1900 considered the skin a barometer for the body's health. Dry skin or rather dry cells in the skin was an indication of a dry body or dry cells in the body. For them this was considered a sign of an unhealthy body with the risk of associated illnesses.

These days the doctors do not use the skin in the same way to judge the health condition any longer, but they use blood tests instead to determine the health status and still most of us have dry skin and body due to lack of the lipids Omega 3 and vitamin A and D.

So what can we do to get more of the healthy lipids into our cells in the skin and the other trillions of cells in the body?

To heal dry skin and body is not as difficult to achieve as you might think it is as long as you follow the method discovered by one doctor in biochemistry in the USA in the early 1940s. He studied illnesses of the metabolism and lipid metabolism with marine oil. With his study he tried to find a method to obtain the lipids Omega 3 and vitamin A & D to prevent illnesses associated with the lack of these healthy lipids. With his method or process to obtain the lipids you can both feel and see the improvement in your skin after a relative short period of time. Before we look into the process to obtain the healthy lipids into the cells of the skin and body let us first try to understand why we, these days, are getting much less of the lipids Omega 3 and vitamin D than previous generations.

As soon as we understand how our modern way of life have influenced our digestion, absorption and transport of the essential fatty acid Omega 3 and the oil soluble vitamin D in the body, compared to previous generations, it should be easier to understand why we get dry skin and body these days.

With this knowledge, it should also be easier to understand what you need to do to obtain a healthy level of Omega 3 and vitamin D together with the other oil soluble vitamins to correct or avoid dry skin and body, and the associated illnesses. With this information your starting question could be:

What changes have we made to our way of living compared to previous generations which give us a lack of the essential fatty acids Omega 3 and the oil soluble vitamin D?

Old medical studies on the lipid metabolism of Omega 3 and vitamin A & D.

Dry skin and body is nothing new as doctors back in the early years of 1900 discovered the same problems with their patients as we are noticing and discovering mostly on our own these days. At that time the doctor considered the body as a functional unit or organism and the skin was considered the barometer for the body`s health. For them, the living skin was the best part of the body to study many important health problems. Dry skin was looked upon as an unhealthy body with the risk of various illnesses caused by the lack of the important lipids.

During the same period different food and soil related studies were initiated in different Western countries to try to understand and learn more what was required to stay healthy. With these important studies the discoveries of the various vitamins, minerals, enzymes and the different oil soluble vitamins and the essential fatty acid Omega 3 and other lipids were discovered.

After the discovery of the oil soluble vitamin A and D and the essential fatty acid Omega 3 in Cod liver oil and the understanding that these lipids were necessary for good health studies on illnesses of the metabolism and lipid metabolism increased i.e. studies related to the physical and chemical processes that occur inside the body and cells to maintain life.

It was soon understood by the doctors the important lipids in the food were not easy to digest and utilize correctly by the cells in the skin and body. This could easily be seen by the increase in the number of patients with dry skin and body and associated illnesses. As far as I understand the lipid metabolism is even today considered as a very complex process in the body, but very little research, if any, is performed and made available in this important area of health.

Back in the early years of the 1900, without a modern pharmaceutical industry, a doctor was still relative free to investigate healing options on his own. This freedom contributed probably a lot to the number of natural health discoveries made during the early years of the 1900. This was the period which resulted in the discovery of the important lipids we know today with the names of the oil soluble vitamin A, D, E, K and the essential fatty acids Omega 3 and 6 together with all the other vitamins, minerals and enzymes.

With the discovery of the oil soluble vitamin D in 1922 the healing power of the sun know since the days of Hippocrates, known as the father of medicine, who lived approx. 2300 years ago, was finally understood. Some doctors started to utilize the sun for the treatment of difficult skin related illnesses, but with the development of a modern pharmaceutical industry in the 1950s after WW2 such treatments were gradually stopped, not because it did not work, but because new doctors were not educated or did not have any interest in this type of natural medicine.

After the discovery of the essential fatty acid Omega 3 in Cod liver oil in 1933, one doctor in biochemistry at a university in the USA decided to study illnesses of the metabolism and lipid metabolism. With his study he wanted to find out what was required for the important lipids to reach the cells in the skin and body to heal and prevent dry skin and body and the associated illnesses. For his study of lipid metabolism he used marine oil or Cod liver oil known to be rich in the important lipids Omega 3 and vitamin D and the other oil soluble vitamins.

With his research, the doctor discovered that very little of the important lipids in marine oil or food rich in these lipids would reach the cells in the skin and body with the normal method of eating and drinking. The doctor discovered the water or any other watery drink during the meal would influence the digestive process of the important lipids and reduce the lipid transport into the cells of the skin and body. Instead a very high percentage of the important lipids consumed with the food would end up in the liver with very little health benefit for the cells in the skin and body. This is the main reason for dry cells in the skin and body. When no water or any other watery drinks were mixed with the food rich in lipids, he discovered the lipids Omega 3 and vitamin A & D in the food would be able to bypass the liver and reach the cells in the skin and body to heal the dry cells in the skin and body.

His discovery represented a complete new understanding regarding the transport of the lipids Omega 3 and oil soluble vitamins in the body compared to the normal medical understanding. He discovered why people got dry skin and body and the associated illnesses. He discovered also how people could obtain a healthy level of Omega 3 and vitamin A & D to heal and prevent dry skin and body. It seems few doctors were interested or understood the importance of his discovery. Perhaps the introduction of the new chemical medicine by the new pharmaceutical industry at more or less the same time was considered more important than the old food related medicine? Unfortunately his discovery was soon forgotten by most people except for one person in search for a cure against arthritis, who understood the importance of his discovery to heal arthritis.

In addition to the discovery of the influence of water on the lipids in the food the doctor discovered also some additional emulsification processes or break down processes for the lipids. These additional emulsification processes would almost double the lipids to be absorbed and transported into the cells of the skin and body.

One emulsification process or break down process to give high lipid transport of Omega 3 and vitamin A & D into the cells of the skin and body was based on warm homemade soups. He discovered warm homemade soups would act as an emulsifying process for the lipids. The homemade soup would help to bring a much higher percentage of the lipids to the cells in the skin and body as long as no water was consumed with the meal rich in lipids. Different homemade soups where tried i.e. soups with fish, beef, chicken, and vegetables. He discovered all the homemade soups gave the same high emulsifying process for the marine oil or food rich in these lipids, but the soups had to be homemade.

The doctor discovered tinned or canned soups did not manage to emulsify the lipids and could not be used to increase the level of Omega 3 or vitamin D from food rich in these lipids.

He discovered also whole milk or normal full fat milk would also act as an emulsifying process for the marine oil or food rich in these lipids. Low fat milk where the fat had been removed did not manage to emulsify the lipids in the marine oil and gave no healing improvements of dry skin.

Another drink, which could also act as an emulsification process of the lipids was fresh orange juice. The fresh orange juice had to be free from pulp or fibres. The orange juice had to be cleaned through a fine mesh or cloth to remove all the pulp and fibres. Without removing all the pulp and fibre the lipid penetration into the skin would be much less. He discovered also that canned or processed concentrated orange juice did not work, at all.

With his research he discovered water or any other watery drink during the meal, which at the time had become normal for most people, would cause a very large reduction of the lipids Omega 3 and vitamin A & D entering the skin compared to having the same meal without any watery drink. To obtain more lipid penetration into the skin, which was used as a measuring point for the lipid penetration into the cells in the body the doctor discovered it was necessary to avoid water or any other watery drink with the food. Instead the water should be consumed 10 minutes or more before the food. This would enable the water to leave the stomach before the arrival of the food. The meal should also be without water or any other watery drink for a period of 3 hours after the food. This avoidance of any watery drink during and after the meal would enable the digestion to complete without any interference of water.

Homemade soups or room tempered or warm whole milk with the meal, without water or any other watery drink would almost double the Omega 3 and vitamin A & D penetration into the cells of the skin and body. With this added emulsification process up to 95 % of the available lipids in the marine oil or food rich in these lipids would reach the cells in the skin and body.

Room tempered water or any other room tempered watery drink with the same food, without soup or with soup, would reduce the lipid penetration into the skin to approximately 20% of the available lipids.

Cold water or water with ice with the meal, which were popular, would reduce the absorption rate of the lipids from the food into the skin much further with the absorption down to close to zero or 5 % of the available lipids in the food.

Based on his research he established the following percentage estimates of lipid penetration of Omega 3 and vitamin D and the other lipids into the skin from marine oil or other food rich in these lipids. From his estimates of lipid penetration into the skin with various types of lipid meals with Omega 3 and vitamin A & D you will see water or any other watery drink which he named as an oil-free beverage would drastically reduce the lipid penetration into the skin and body, with all types of meals.

- Lipid meal with soup and no water or other oil-free beverages=95% lipid penetration=maximum.
- Lipid meal with room tempered or warm milk during the meal and no water=95%=maximum.

- Lipid meal and no soup and no room tempered or warm milk and no water =50% of maximum.

As soon as water or an oil-free beverage was consumed with the meal or after the meal within the 3 hour digestive period, the doctor discovered the lipid penetration of the important lipids into the cells in the skin would drop considerably.

- Lipid meal with water=20% of maximum lipid penetration.
- Lipid meal with soup and water=20% of maximum lipid penetration.
- Lipid meal and ice cold water=5% of maximum lipid penetration.
- Lipid meal with soup and ice cold water=5% of maximum lipid penetration.

To obtain a level of 50 % of the available lipids Omega 3 and vitamin D and the other lipids into the cells in the skin and body, he discovered it was necessary to avoid water or any other watery drink with the meal. Instead the water or any other watery drink should be consumed 10 minutes or more before the food with no watery drinks for up to 3 hours after the food to complete the digestion without any influence of water or any other watery drink.

To obtain a maximum level of the available lipids with 95 % from the food it was necessary to add a homemade soup with the meal without water or use room tempered or warm milk with the food.

As soon as water or any other watery drink was introduced with the meals the lipid level from the food reaching the cells in the skin would drop drastically. With cold watery drinks the lipid level reaching the cells in the skin and body would be reduced to almost zero or 5 %.

The difference between the maximum and the minimum absorption rates of the important lipids Omega 3 and vitamin A & D from the same type of meal rich in lipids, are almost 20 times! Without following this simple rule of separating food and water or any other watery drink, which he defined as an oil-free beverage, during the meal, there would be very little of the lipids available in the food which would reach the cells of the skin and body. The lack of the important lipids would cause the cells in the skin and body to dry out over time with a risk of associated illnesses.

In other words the doctor discovered it is not enough to eat good fatty fish food or other good food containing the essential fatty acid Omega 3 and the oil soluble vitamin D to obtain a healthy level of these important lipids, but you need also to know when to drink your water or any other watery drink. In addition you need also to add a homemade soup or room tempered or warm whole milk to the meal. The homemade soup or the milk is required to emulsify and release the last 45 % of the lipids in the food.

Not drinking water with the meal, but instead drinking water 10-30 minutes before the meal and approximately 3 hours after the meal to improve health have for some families in certain countries been known for long time if not hundreds of years. For them the food and water separation was a normal habit, but over time it seems to have been forgotten for various reasons.

During the last 100 years or so we have seen large change in our societies with large movement of people from the country side to the cities with a gradual change to smaller families. The invention of the automobile influenced the transport to and from work for everyone and with this major change a lot of the old eating and drinking habits changed too. These days it is normal for many people living in the cities to eat at restaurants almost daily, but this habit did not exist hundred years ago. Food preparations and eating habits at home have also changed to a large extent.

Another doctor in biochemistry in Germany who studied oils and fats and their metabolism in the cells in the body over very long period of time in the 1940s and 50s discovered also the oils would need to go through an emulsification or mixing process before the oil could be absorbed and distributed via the blood circulation and the capillaries into the cells in the body. With the emulsification process of the oil the doctor achieved a correct metabolism at the cellular level with the result of detoxification of old fats and healing at the cellular level.

The study of oils and fats and their metabolism in the cells of the human body seems to be a very time consuming study. This might be the reason why there has not been any new large scale study undertaken by any university on the subject to guide people to eat and drink more healthy to help to avoid or reduce the many illnesses caused by the wrong metabolism of oils and fat.

Until a new study on the lipid metabolism in the human body is undertaken and published you can however still utilize the old information on the lipid metabolism to heal your dry skin and body with a healthy level of Omega 3 and vitamin A & D. Dry skin, according to the doctors back in the early 1900, was the same as not having a healthy level of the important lipids in the cells in the body.

The good thing with a healthy level of the essential fatty acid Omega 3 and the oil soluble vitamin A & D is that you can see and feel it with your soft and moist skin.

With this information you should now also be able to make a good guess why we over time get dry skin and body and other health related problems much earlier in life than before.

Changes in eating habits and food sources cause lack of the lipids Omega 3 and vitamin D.

Eating and drinking habits.

The doctor who studied lipid metabolism with marine oil to obtain a healthy level of the essential fatty acid Omega 3 and the oil soluble vitamin A and D, discovered with his research that it is not enough to select and to eat wild fatty fish or other food rich in the lipids to obtain the healthy lipids. You need also to know when to drink or not to drink with your food and to use homemade soups to bring out more of the healthy lipids from the marine oil or food rich in lipids.

Even if we should obtain and eat wild fatty fish or other good food rich in Omega 3 and vitamin D, and apply the correct cooking to preserve the healthy lipids, several times a week, for a long time most of us would still end up with dry skin, hair and body. The water or any other watery drink we drink during the meal will prevent the lipids to reach the cells in the skin.

The incorrect use of water or any other watery drink, mainly due to lack of digestive knowledge of the healthy lipids, is the main reason why we end up with dry skin, hair and body. Previous generations did not have this digestive knowledge either, but most people at that time had a different habit of drinking water with their food.

With his study the doctor discovered you have to drink your water 10 minutes before your food, to enable the water to leave the stomach before the arrival of the food. No water or any other watery drink should be consumed during the meal for a period of approximately 3 hours after the meal. This is to enable the digestion to complete without the interruption of any watery drink. Without following this simple method of separating water or any other watery drink from the food very little of the important lipids in the food would be utilized correctly in the body. The same will apply to the use of marine oil supplements known to be rich in these important lipids.

Doctors who studied food metabolism and health much earlier discovered also the influence of water on the digestion of the food. These doctors focused most of their study on the protein and carbohydrate metabolism and had no interest or knowledge of the oil soluble vitamins and the essential fatty acids or lipids. Some of them must have discovered water's influence on the digestion of the food. More recent studies on water and health, by one doctor who lived in the USA, confirms that your digestive system will be supported by the water, if the water is consumed on an empty stomach approximately 30 minutes before the food with no water for 3 hours after the food.

These old and new digestive studies of water and health confirms that it is not only the essential fatty acid Omega 3 and the oil soluble vitamin D and other lipids which will be absorbed wrongly with the wrong timing of the water or any other watery drink, but your entire digestive system will be affected with the risk of more nutrients than the important lipids in the food can be wasted.

To understand how previous generations avoided having problems with water and the break down process or emulsification process of the food to obtain a high absorption rate of the healthy lipids Omega 3 and vitamin D with the other lipids and other healthy nutrients from the food let us briefly refresh some of the previous information.

The digestive system and the cells in the skin and body respond differently to the marine oil with Omega 3 and vitamin A & D or food rich in these lipids with water than without water. To obtain a correct absorption and transport of the lipids into the cells in the skin and body the lipids had to enter the digestive process without water. To obtain a high healthy level of the lipids the food had to be consumed without water or any watery drink. Water or any other watery drink had to be consumed at least 10 minutes before the food and no watery drink should enter the digestive system for another period of approximately 3 hours. By following this water rule the oil or the lipids would be digested correctly so that approximately 50 % of the available lipids in the marine oil or food rich in the lipids would reach the cells in the skin and body. By having an additional homemade soup or room tempered or warm whole milk with the meal up to 95 % of the available lipids Omega 3 and vitamin A & D in the meal would be digested, absorbed, transported, distributed and utilized correctly in the cells of the skin and body.

If cold water or any cold watery drink was entered into the digestive process with the food a very small percentage of the important lipids with only 5% of the available lipids would reach the cells in the skin and body. Somehow the lipids got caught by another organ in the body!

The correct metabolism of the lipids Omega 3 and vitamin A & D in the body can somehow be compared to a cook handling various ingredients to create a special good meal. The cook need more than the right ingredients to produce a good meal. The cook requires also knowledge about the cooking temperatures and when to mix the ingredients together or emulsify the ingredients to achieve the expected end result. Without this special knowledge the end result of the meal will be different each time even if the same ingredients are used each time.

If we use the above mentioned information and take the time to study how previous generations lived and worked we will discover the majority of the people prepared the food slightly different compared to what we do today. We will also discover that a lot of people had a habit of eating and drinking which is slightly different from the habit we have today.

So what are the main differences in the food preparations and eating habits between previous generations and us which can have such a large impact on the correct absorption of the healthy lipids Omega 3 and vitamin D?

A study of old kitchen ovens and kitchen utensils in the museums will give us the answers to the cooking methods used hundreds of years ago or even further back in time. In the museums we will find large pots which were used for cooking the food. We will also find large cast iron ovens or stoves for wood or coal firing with one or two cooking plates or holes for the pots.

From the study of the cast iron ovens or stoves with only one or two cooking plates or holes for the big pots we can easily make assumptions on the type of food most families used. One pot would most likely contain a thick soup or stew with vegetables with something else such as chicken, fish or meat added to the pot, i.e. a good homemade soup.

Homemade soup meals were probably served every day of the week or at least most days of the week in most families. This method of cooking and serving was relatively easy to do on the type of oven or stove available at the time. With a thick soup or stew in the pot the food could be kept lightly warm so that the meal could be heated up and served within 10 minutes or more after the people arrived at home to eat or rest. With a soup or stew, we can also assume that there would be very little drinking during the meal or after the meal.

We can also assume a majority of people would come home to eat and rest. Before the automobile they would walk a lot or use bicycles or any other physical means of transport. With this natural physical exercise we can also assume it would be normal for people to be thirsty when they arrived home. Most likely they would drink their water, as soon as they came in the door. After the water they would do other things before they had their warm food, i.e. they would more or less always obtain a 10 minutes or more waiting period between the water drink and the warm food without even thinking about it. We can also assume the food would consist of a homemade soup out of a large pot. Before we got piped water into the houses the water had to be brought home from a central water supply or natural stream. We can assume the water would be kept indoors close to the entrance door. At the door, the water would be easy to reach and drink when people arrived home for food and rest. The water would always be room tempered. The invention of the refrigerator with ice cold water or other drinks is also a relative new invention.

Before the cast iron oven or stove period, the food cooking was mostly arranged from a fire place with the use of one pot. The pot used to hang in the centre of the fireplace. Again a heavy homemade soup or stew was most likely used for most of the meals. Before the copper or iron pot period, clay pots were used to store and heat the food. Homemade soups have been used to feed people for thousands of years.

So what is so special with these old food preparations and eating and water drinking habits which have changed so completely in the Western world over the last few hundred years or so?

As mentioned earlier, the doctor discovered with his research on the lipid metabolism with marine oil to obtain Omega 3 and vitamin A & D or food rich in these lipids the water or any other watery drink with the meal reduced the lipid penetration into the cells of the skin. He discovered also the marine oil required an additional process for the correct break down or emulsification of the lipids. Without this emulsification process very little of the important lipids would reach the cells in the skin, which at that time was used as a measuring point for the lipid penetration to the cells in the body.

It was discovered the additional emulsifier could be homemade soups or room tempered or warm whole milk as both acted as an emulsifier for the lipids in the food. With this emulsifier a very high percentage of the lipids would reach the cells in the skin and the body, as long as no water was part of the digestive process.

The doctor discovered also ice cold water or other ice cold drinks consumed with the meals would reduce the lipid distribution and transport to the cells in the skin and body close to zero or only 5 %. The low 5 % rate should be compared to the high lipid distribution rate of approximately 95 % obtained with a meal with homemade soups or room tempered or warm whole milk, with no water. By adding a homemade soup to the meal there is an almost 20 times higher penetration rate of the available lipids in the food into the cells of the skin compared to a meal with a cold drink! Water and especially a cold watery drink reduce very much the correct absorption of the important lipids.

With his research he discovered water and oils or lipids do not mix. This chemical phenomenon applies to the water entering the human stomach together with the oil or lipids as well as anywhere else. No matter how hard you try, water and oil will not mix, without the application of an emulsification process which is a combined chemical and physical process.

These days it has become normal to drink water with all the meals or some of the many watery drinks which are available in an ever increasing supply with cold or ice cold soda drinks, cola drinks, sparkling water, tea, coffee, espresso, cappuccino, beer, wine, etc, with the meal, during the meal or after the meal. Water or some other oil-free beverage is normally always on the table whenever or wherever we sit down to eat, but this was not so normal back in time as there were no need for it. The use of the many watery drinks with food has become a habit and with this habit you lose most of the important and healthy lipids Omega 3 and vitamin D!

In the old days, before the automobile, people had to walk, cycle or use carriages with horses to move around. With this physical exercise most people would be thirsty when they arrived home. Water which was a normal drink was normally kept inside at the entrance door so it would be easy to reach and it would be room tempered. The majority of the people at that time would normally drink their water when they were thirsty as soon as they came home to eat and rest. After they had stopped their thirst they would wash or do other things while the food would be heated. With this normal habit of drinking their water when they were thirsty they would most of the days obtain 10 minutes or even more time between the water and the food. As they were not thirsty it was no need to drink water during the meal. A rest after the meal for a few hours, due to long working hours was probably also very normal for a lot of people in those days.

With this normal way of living, eating and consuming water when thirsty a large percentage of the population would not have a problem with the wrong combination of food and water or any other watery drink, most of the times.

I learned from my present wife's mother, who is German and live in Hamburg and reached the good age of 87 in 2010 and is still with good health, that in her parents' house it was normal not to drink water when eating. As children, they were told not to drink water with the meals to obtain a better digestion of the food to improve their health. Their parents had learned it from their parents and so on. For them it was normal not to drink when eating, but instead they would normally drink 10-30 minutes before the food and approx. 3 hours after the food. In this way they somehow knew or had been told that they would get a better digestion of the food and more nutrients from the food and a better health.

According to my wife's mother her parents followed this way of separating food and drink most of the time and the only exceptions were celebrations.

With this small separation of the food and the water the people would obtain a correct digestion, transport and distribution of the healthy lipids in the food to the cells in the skin and body with a correct metabolism. Should the meal also include a homemade soup as a starter, which was often the case in the old days, a high amount of lipids with up to 95 % of the available lipids in the food would reach the cells in the skin and body.

Gradually over time with the small changes in our way of living we lost without knowing it the important separation of food and water and the equal important homemade soups which had kept previous generations, for thousands of years relatively healthy, probably without knowing it. For them it was the most natural way or habit to eat and drink.

Today, this habit or method of eating and drinking to protect good health has unfortunately been lost to most people.

The first major change of living, eating and drinking habits for a large percentage of the population in the Western world started much earlier than the introduction of the automobile for transport. It started mainly with the industrial revolution 1760-1850 or up to the early 1900. During this period a large number of people started to move from the country side into the cities to find better opportunities. Rickets or bone problems became a large public health problem in some countries. The lack of exposure to the sun was considered the cause of it, but most likely both the lack of exposure to the sun and the new and changed habit of drinking water with the food, was a combined reason for the widespread illness. The illness was brought under control with improved food sources with Omega 3 and vitamin A and D, but new research has concluded that rickets is one of the easiest illnesses to cure with a relative small increase of the healthy lipids from the food. This is probably why not many people get rickets today.

New research by different universities both in the USA and Europe have come to the conclusion that we need a much higher level of vitamin D to prevent and cure many of the more serious illnesses we are facing today. The level of vitamin D they consider preventive for most of the serious illnesses is more than 10 times the current daily recommended level of vitamin D!

Perhaps this high level of vitamin D was the level of vitamin D, previous generations managed to obtain with their outdoor work with their natural exposure to the sun without sun protection, reasonable diet with homemade soups and their natural separation of water and food in most of their meals?

Serious illness associated with a lack of the healthy lipids Omega 3 and vitamin D seems to have started to increase during the early years of the 1900 with a much more rapid increase since the 1960s. Since the 1960s we have also experienced a very large change in the eating and drinking habits for a very large percentage of the people in Western world and it seems this change is accelerating. This change with the eating and drinking habits are now gradually also being adopted by people in the rest of the world who has also started to move from the countryside into the cities for better opportunities.

Food is lacking Omega 3 and vitamin D.

In addition to the changes we have introduced to our food habits over the last hundred years or so, we have also over the last 50 years got another perhaps equal important food related issue to consider when eating food containing fish, eggs and meat, i.e. the main food sources used by many people to try to obtain the essential fatty acid Omega 3, and the oil soluble vitamin D plus the other healthy lipids and nutrients.

For the fish and the animals to produce a meat with a normal level of the essential fatty acid Omega 3 and the oil soluble vitamin D the fish and the animals need to eat their natural diet. This is not the case any longer for most of our fish, meat, and eggs we buy in the super market these days. The fish, meat and egg farming, which have been developed over the last 40 years or so to obtain low priced products, has changed this.

Some of our fat fish, like the pink salmon, is most likely a farmed fish these days due to the high cost to obtain wild salmon. The same applies to most of our beef, chicken and eggs. Most food is from grain feed hens or animals with little or no access to their natural diet. Such food is also containing other questionable ingredients linked to their medication to increase their weight and to keep them healthy in cramped feed lots, but as this is not related to the lack of the essential fatty acid Omega 3 and the oil soluble vitamin D I will not bring it up here.

Without a natural diet our farmed fish and grain feed animals, being organic or not organic, have very little natural Omega 3, and vitamin D. Most of the food is instead high in the lipid Omega 6 due to the grain feeding. Our bodies do not need too much of the lipid Omega 6, even if Omega 6 is part of the essential fatty acids required by the body. Normally Omega 6 and Omega 3 exist in a balance in the food and body, but with food lacking Omega 3 and instead have a high level of Omega 6 there will be an imbalance between these two essential fatty acids in the body when we eat this type of food. This imbalance between the two important essential fatty acids is a fairly new area of health and there is not much medical research available regarding the imbalance between these 2 essential fatty acids, caused by the new and unnatural diet for the animals.

Previous generations did not have this problem to think about as their fish and animals lived wild or free range with natural food from the sea and the fields. With natural food the Omega 3 to Omega 6 ratio in the food stayed within a natural band of Omega 3 to Omega 6 of 1 to 1. These days, this relationship has shifted drastically into much higher ratios like 1 to 10 or 1 to 20 or even with much higher ratios where the lipid Omega 6 is dominating.

Another food related issue of concern is our large selection of tinned or canned food, these days. From the research made by the doctor on the lipid metabolism with marine oil with Omega 3 and vitamin A and D, he discovered tinned or canned soups, which had become popular at the time, did not have the ability to emulsify the lipids in the food or bring the important lipids into the cells of the skin, as he could do with homemade soup. With this discovery I guess we have to conclude that tinned or canned food is practically without healthy lipids even if the food inside the tin or can should contain the lipids. Something seems to have happened to the food content during the canning process. After all, the canning process was invented back in 1810 for the army. It was invented as a method to prevent the food to be spoilt and to provide food to the soldiers during military campaigns when it was difficult to transport fresh food. Since then, the canning process has improved, but as far as I know there has not been any research performed to check if the cells in the body are able to benefit from the various lipids and some other ingredients present in the food. Perhaps this type of canned food should be considered more as an emergency food only, which was the original idea by the army?

One food source, rich in nutrients, not many people are aware of any longer is the use of the liver and the kidneys of free range or wild animals, which previous generations utilized for food. The liver of any animal has for hundreds if not thousands of years been recognized as the storage point for nutrients and a good food source. The liver and the kidneys were considered by previous generations as a health food, but somehow it has disappeared more and more over the last 30-40 years. With the new medication and artificial food used in farming these days, it is for the better, but for previous generations, in the days with free range animals, the liver and the kidneys were considered a good source of various healthy nutrients.

The sunshine vitamin, vitamin D.

Previous generations used the sun and the healing power from the sun to improve health much more than most of us do today. The sun's healing power has been well known to the broad society since the days of Hippocrates, who lived approximately 350 BC or approximately 2300 years ago and is known as the father of modern Western medicine, or even before his time. At that time they did not know the sun generated vitamin D in the skin, but they still understood, from experience, the sun was important for good health. Today we know the healing power of the sun is coming from the important oil soluble vitamin D generated in the skin by the rays of the sun, but still most people these days do the best to block out the sun's rays with various sun blockers.

From my recent visits to a small museum displaying old terracotta figures of people from Latin America, I could see Terracotta figures of ladies from Costa Rica dating back to approx. 300BC to 200AD. The ladies were wearing what I would call modern bikinis or G-strings only and no bra, but the breasts were decorated and matching the decoration on the bikini. These approximately 2000 years old ladies, immortalised in the Terracotta figures, were obvious enjoying the healing power of the sun.

Another modern development to consider is also the move of more and more people into the cities. Previous generations lived more in the country side and had many opportunities to utilize the sun's healing rays by working outdoors or being outdoors. These days with more people living in apartments in the cities they might have little opportunities to experience the natural healing power of the sun. With this change the healing power of the sun has been lost for a large percentage of the population.

Eating habits and food changes since the industrial revolution.

With all these small, but very important changes in how we live, work, transport, eat and drink compared to previous generations most of us have lost the healthy intake of the essential fatty acid Omega 3 and what seems to be the equal important oil soluble vitamin D.

The first real major change in the eating and drinking habits for a large percentage of the Western population happened during the industrial revolution when a large number of people moved from the country side into the cities to live and work. More recently we got another much larger change with the introduction of the automobile in the early years of 1900 up to the 1950s which caused large changes in the way people moved to and from work. After the WW2 or the 1950s we had another large move of people from the country side into the cities. With all these movements of people, people changed gradual their old eating and drinking habits at home. The introduction of canned or tinned food, originally invented as a food for the army at war, increased. People saw the convenience with the tinned food as it was easy to store at home and fast to prepare. The introduction of glass bottles helped also to increase the consumption of the new watery drinks with food, both during and after the meal. The invention of the fridge gave us cold drinks. The eating out at restaurants started also to increase for more and more people.

Later on in the Western part of the world, we got new food sources with the introduction of feed lots for the animals with the gradual introduction of grain feeding of the animals, good for fattening, instead of free roaming animals eating natural grass in the country side. The fish farming industry did more or less the same and ended up with hardly any natural food for the fish production, but they are still producing nice looking fish. The industrial farmed beef, eggs and fish have low levels of natural Omega 3 and vitamin D and other lipids compared to wild animals and fish.

More recently we have got the sun lotions or sun blockers, blocking out the healthy sun rays and vitamin D, used by previous generations for thousands of years. To protect the skin against the healthy sun rays people are instead plastering their skin with various toxic ingredients which are part of the sunscreen lotions and other skin lotions. These toxic ingredients are penetrating the skin layers and are finding their way into the lymphatic system and the blood circulation ending up in the spleen, the kidneys and the liver where they over time together with other toxins can be the cause of malfunctions in these organs.

The latest fad or addiction affecting the correct absorption and transport of the healthy lipids into the cells of the skin and body is the new consumption of the many coffee and soft drinks by the young generation with each meal! Not only do the drinks prevent the correct digestion and transport of the healthy lipids into the cells, but the drinks cause also acid blood and body and bring lots of toxins into the cells and the organs.

In other words you can say it took us approximately 100 years or so to complete the reduction of the healthy and essential fatty acid Omega 3 and the oil soluble vitamin D in our diet and food sources. The result of this gradual change with lack of the important lipids can now be seen in the increase of illnesses. Previously it was considered normal with illnesses at high age, but these days some of the old age related illnesses are slowly moving down to the younger generation.

The following list gives a brief overview of the main developments during the last 100 years or so which represents the main changes and causes responsible for the reduced intake of the important and essential fatty acid Omega 3 and the oil soluble vitamin D.

- The move of people to the cities into apartments from the sunny country side.
- The mixing of food and water in each meal instead of drinking water first as our ancestors.
- The introduction and the increased use of canned or tinned food.
- The loss of the homemade soups in the meals.
- The introduction of bottled and canned drinks.
- The invention of the fridge which gave us cold drinks, which eliminates almost all the lipids.
- Farmed fish, meat and eggs feed an unnatural diet, producing low levels of Omega 3, and vitamin D with high level of Omega 6, which started for full in the 1960s.
- Other food changes, which also reduce the intake of Omega 3 and vitamin D.

- The avoidance of the healthy sun with sun blocking lotions.
- More people started to eat at cafes and restaurants with a questionable nutritional value.
- The increased use of highly refined and processed acid food with hardly any nutritional value.
- The new addiction to the many acid coffee and soft drinks by the young generation.

Previous generations who lived and worked mostly in the country side and came home to eat and rest did not have much health problems related to the lack of what we now call essential fatty acid Omega 3 with EPA & DHA and the oil soluble vitamin D as long as they had access to some good food sources. Yes, they had illnesses, but they were different and most of them were solved over time with improved diet, clean drinking water and proper sanitation.

Today, even with a very large selection of what many people consider good food sources rich in Omega 3 and vitamin D, it seems that we have managed to reduce our intake of the natural occurring Omega 3 and vitamin D to a level which seems not to support our health in the long run.

If you have dry skin or hair and need to apply lotions to your skin and hair to keep it moist and soft and you think you eat well perhaps you now understand why you get so little of the important lipids Omega 3 and the oil soluble vitamin A and D from your fish, beef, eggs and other food sources?

Dry skin and body with all the under the skin health problems seems to increase and has become a relatively new and large health problem in the Western world. It will also spread to other parts of the world with the large movement of people from the countryside into the cities who will also adopt new habits of drinking water or any watery drink with the food and the avoidance of the sun.

One dentist with a special interest in health, who travelled around the world for some extended period of time in the 1920s and 30s and studied health of primitive and isolated populations noticed, already at that time, the good health of the isolated populations started to decline for each generation as soon as they started to adopt more to the Western diet high in refined food.

Food sources with Omega-3 and vitamin D.

Previous generations had many natural food sources available to them to obtain their essential fatty acids Omega 3 and the oil soluble vitamin D, even if they did not know the name or their existence at that time. Some families started also long time ago to collect information on healthy food and passed this collection of food and health knowledge to their children. The children passed it on to their children so it stayed in the families over hundreds of years if not longer. The families somehow knew what type of food to eat to stay reasonably healthy. Some families knew also the combination of water and food together was not good for health. They had learned to separate the water and food. They would drink their water when thirsty before the food with no water during the meal up to 3 hours after the food. By following this old collected family food and water drinking knowledge they knew, like their parents and their grandparents that they would obtain more of the important nutrients from the food to stay healthy.

These days, this valuable information on health through the food and water has been lost to most people.

Instead we get most of our food from fish farms, chicken farms, egg farms, meat farms. In these farms the fish and animals are being feed a diet which is completely different from the diet of wild fish and grass feed animals. The result of this is a food with a questionable level of the natural essential fatty acid Omega 3 and Omega 6 and the oil soluble vitamin D. The food from the food farms is then canned or tinned into all types and forms of processed and refined food, which is another much more questionable food source these days.

With the type of food industry we have today it is not so easy to find food with the natural and healthy level of Omega 3 and vitamin D.

So what shall you do?

The cells in your body need the essential fatty acid Omega 3 and the oil soluble vitamin D plus other lipids and nutrients to stay healthy and function properly. This is nothing new and was discovered already in the early years of the 1900 with the discovery of the vitamins, minerals, enzymes and the essential fatty acids.

From the research by the doctor who studied illnesses of the metabolism and lipid metabolism with marine oil with the aim to find a method to obtain the important lipids Omega 3 and vitamin A and D, we know that it is not sufficient to eat good food to obtain the important lipids if we drink water or any other watery drink with the food. We need to plan our water drinking. We need to change our drinking habit! We should stop drinking water or any other watery drink with our food and instead drink water 10 minutes or more before the food and 3 hours after the food. With this change of habit you can increase the absorption rate of the healthy lipids from approximately 5 % to 50 % of the available lipids in the food, as previously explained. This is equivalent to a 10 times increase from what you would normally obtain from your food with a cold drink. Should you also add a homemade soup to the meal with no water you can even reach close to 95 % of the available lipids in the food which is almost a 20 times increase compared to having the food with a cold drink.

If you still feel that you want to try to find good food sources with natural Omega 3 and vitamin D, the following could be a general guide;

- Wild fresh fish from cold sea water with a natural diet, such as mackerel, salmon, herrings, sardines, trout, tuna or the roe or liver of the Cod fish from the cold waters and some other fish types. Wild fish from warm sea waters have less Omega 3 and vitamin D, compared to wild fish from cold sea water, but such fish, to obtain the important lipids, is better than no fish.

- Meat from animals having access to fresh natural grass and plants from the fields.
- Eggs, but the eggs should come from free-range or free roaming hens with a natural free range diet. The natural diet is required by the hens to produce natural Omega 3 and vitamin D. Grain feed animals will have more of the lipid Omega 6 than Omega 3.
- Some fresh nuts, like Walnuts, Hazel nuts, Brazil nuts and some other nuts.
- Fresh green vegetables. Avocados.
- Avoid canned or tinned products.
- Avoid vegetable oils rich in the lipid Omega 6.

With this food selection, with natural wild and fresh food, you should have a good chance to obtain a good level of the lipids Omega 3 and vitamin D from the food, but remember you need also to prepare the food correctly and you should not drink water or any other watery drink with your food. The important lipids in the food are heat sensitive and should not be burnt or oxidized in the heating process. For this reason avoid frying the food with high heat and avoid deep frying in vegetable oils normally rich in Omega 6. Previous generations cooked their food mostly in large pots like a homemade soup or stew. According to the doctor who studied the lipid metabolism the homemade soup will give a high level of the important lipids into the cells in the skin and body, as long as you do not drink water or any other watery with the meal, as previously explained.

If your skin or hair is still dry after 6 months to a year on what you consider a good diet with no water or any other watery drink with your meal, something is wrong, either with your food source or your method of preparing the food.

In the old days when your skin was considered the barometer for your health, dry skin was considered a warning signal that your body was running low on the essential fatty acid Omega 3 and vitamin A and D!

The good thing with a correct and healthy level of the lipids Omega 3 and vitamin A and D in your cells in your skin and body is that you should be able to feel your skin is soft and moist without being oily and without the application of any cream or lotions. With the correct supply of the healthy lipids the natural moisture to the cells is supplied to all the cells from the inside via the blood circulation.

Why is Omega 3 and vitamin D so important?

Omega 3 with the DHA and EPA and Omega 6 are part of a family of essential fatty acids, which the body cannot produce and must obtain from the food. The lipids Omega 3 and 6 together with the oil soluble vitamins A, D, E and K are parts of the cells. They exist in all the trillions of cells in the body. Without their presence at a healthy level the proper functions of all cellular activities in the body will be affected. In other words, they are essential for a healthy body.

The importance of the inclusion and use of good oils, in our daily diet, have been known for a very long time, but the oil soluble vitamin D was first discovered in 1922 and the essential fatty acid Omega 3 was identified in 1933, but it is not until more recently, with new research, that a much wider understanding of their many important functions have been discovered. These days we know the essential fatty acid Omega 3 transport oxygen to the cells in the body and every cell require oxygen for its proper function. We also know Omega 3 and vitamin D help in the detoxification process at the cellular level because of their slightly negative charge expelling toxins with a slightly positive charge.

The DHA (docosahexaenoic acid) and EPA (eicosapentaenoic acid) parts of the Omega 3 are the best known parts and their important health benefits were better understood in the 1970's with studies of the Greenland Inuit tribe, who lived a healthy life on large amount of fat from seafood. These days new research is bringing new awareness and understanding of the importance of the essential fatty acids Omega 3 for our health.

Vitamin D, together with the oil soluble vitamin A, was for a very long time thought to help the growth of bones only, but today with new research, vitamin D is considered to be a very complex oil soluble substance in the cells. It has been discovered vitamin D is also acting as a hormone in many functions and processes in the body. There are also old studies proposing the natural oil soluble vitamin D work more efficient in the body when taken together with the natural oil soluble vitamin A. In some food and marine oil both the oil soluble vitamins A and D exist together.

The exact function of vitamin D with its many hormonal functions is still not fully understood, but what it is known is that vitamin D protect and maintain wellness in the body and treat illnesses.

One of the most recent medical discoveries with the involvement of vitamin D is related to the Nobel Prize in Medicine in 2009 with the discovery of the enzyme Telomerase. The enzyme Telomerase is controlling the biological clock or aging in the DNA via the chromosome telomere. The chromosome telomere is activated by different hormones including vitamin D. When we consider there are hundreds if not thousands of different chemical processes identified in the cells in the body and new ones are discovered, it will probably take some years before the many functions of the oil soluble vitamin D are fully understood.

Vitamin D or the form D 3 which is the active form of vitamin D seems to be generated mostly in the skin by the UVB rays from the sun. The UVB rays are creating biochemical reactions in the cells of the deep layers of the skin where the vitamin D is transformed and transferred into the blood circulation. From the blood circulation via the capillaries the D3 vitamin will reach all the cells in the body.

The sun has also another entry point into the cells in the body than the skin. An entry point most of us do not think about as an entry point. Open eyes, but without glasses. One doctor claimed to have discovered by chance the sunlight entering the eyes without glasses has a much stronger vitamin D effect in the cells than the sun entering the skin without sun protection. It seems the sunlight activate the glands in the brain that control the production of hormones. Remember vitamin D is a hormone. The invention of glasses to improve vision seems to date back to year 1284, in Italy. Since then eye glasses have been used to improve vision and block out sun light. Even normal window glass reduces greatly the sun's full wavelength energy. Plants use the sun's different wavelength energy in a process called photosynthesis to develop and grow. Plants can get a tremendous strength from the sun's wavelength energy, but without sunlight the plant age very fast. The only way to find out if the doctor was right with his prediction that sunlight through the eyes produce vitamin D is to test it out. Stay out in the sunlight without glasses and without getting burnt. Perhaps he was right? I do not know, but in case he was right the vitamin D medicine from the sun is free.

The sunlight has provided the healthy form of vitamin D 3 for thousands of years, but this natural method to obtain vitamin D 3 seems to have been forgotten by many people these days with the wide spread use of sun cream and sun glasses blocking out the UVB rays.

The body generate different types of essential fatty acids, but the essential fatty acids Omega 3 and Omega 6 have to come from the food we eat. The body generate also different types of vitamin D, but the important form of vitamin D is the form D3. Vitamin D3 is normally generated in the skin, by the sun, and exists in certain food sources, but the food sources for vitamin D3 are limited. For this reason vitamin D is added to certain food, and given as supplements, but mostly in the form of D 2 which is not the same as the healthy form D 3.

Dry skin was considered by doctors in the 1940s as a good sign of a dry body. Already at that time they had identified a number of illnesses related to dry skin and body caused by the lack of Omega 3 and vitamin A & D. These days many more illnesses are identified.

According to scientific research lack of these important lipids cause oxidative stress or inflammation at the cellular level.

Should you have dry skin and need to apply cream or skin lotions to keep it moist, a good insurance against this situation and the many forms of illnesses which can develop over time due to the lack of the healthy natural lipids would be to start a supplementation method with Omega 3 and the oil soluble vitamin A and D, the correct and natural way, which is the topic of this book.

The relationship between Omega 3 and Omega 6.

Omega 6 is another essential fatty acid or lipid like Omega 3 which the body needs to obtain from the food we eat. Normally the Omega 6 and the Omega 3 lipids works together in a relationship or have a controlling influence on each other in the body i.e. the function of Omega 6 is somehow controlled by the functions or presence of the Omega 3.

The balance between Omega 6 and Omega 3 is better explained by the functions of each type of essential fatty acids. Omega 3 is considered as an anti-inflammatory essential fatty acid while Omega 6 is considered a pro-inflammatory essential fatty acid i.e. the lipid Omega 6 is there to cause inflammation, for whatever reason.

Too much of the pro-inflammatory lipid Omega 6 cannot be good for health, and this is probably the reason why the lipid Omega 3 is so important.

The lipid Omega 6 is present in food like grain, corn and some vegetable oils such as sunflower, soya, canola or rapeseed etc. Our intake of the lipid Omega 6 which is included in almost any prefabricated food, snacks, etc, has reached a very high level in our food chain today.

The normal relationship between Omega 3 to Omega 6 in the cells in the body should be 1:1 or only slightly higher. These days, a high percentage of the population seems to have reached a ratio between Omega 3 and Omega 6 of up to 1: 10 or 1: 20 or even much higher. The high ratio of Omega 6 is caused by the increased consumption of all types of fast food, processed food, snacks and vegetable oils. The consumption of fish, meat and eggs from food farms utilizing a lot of grain or other ingredients in the feed for the fish and the animals will also increase the ratio of the Omega 6 as this type of food has more Omega 6 than Omega 3.

The imbalance or wrong balance between the two essential fatty acids Omega 3 and Omega 6 is creating a relative new situation in the in the body, as the use of food rich in Omega 6 is relative new. Until there is more medical research and understanding of what the imbalance between the lipids Omega 3 and Omega 6 will have on health it seems to be impossible to say what the imbalance between the two Omegas will bring.

It is however possible to start to make a healthy correction of the imbalance between the two Omegas by increasing the intake or the level of Omega 3 with a supplementation with Omega 3 and vitamin D the natural and correct way which is the topic of this book.

At the same time it can be advisable to try to reduce the consumption of food, vegetable oils and snacks high in the lipids Omega 6.

Early warning signals for lack of the lipids Omega 3 and vitamin A & D.

Some of the early warning signals for lack of the important lipids Omega 3 and vitamin A & D in the cells in the body in addition to dry skin can be the following:

- Flakiness or dryness on the legs.
- Thick, rough or cracked skin on the heels.
- Scales on the elbows and knees.
- Stretch marks on tights and buttocks.
- Small wrinkles as dry skin is the forerunner to wrinkled skin.
- Bad fingernails.
- Dandruff.
- Dry hair.
- Lack of yellow earwax.
- Crusty dirt in the corners of the eyes in the morning.
- Long waiting time on the toilet.
- Itching.

Other more serious signals for the lack of the important lipids can be found under next chapter **"Illnesses linked to lack of the lipids Omega 3 and vitamin D"** where the focus is directed towards problems identified with the possible lack of Omega 3 and vitamin D. It seems the body has more problems to obtain a healthy level of these two important lipids from the food than some of the other oil soluble vitamins. For this reason serious illnesses related to lack of the oil soluble vitamin A and the other oil soluble vitamins seem to be rare today.

Old studies on the oil soluble vitamins found that vitamin D needs vitamin A to function properly in the body and in certain natural food such as marine oil, both vitamin D and A exists together.

The good thing with a healthy level of the important lipids is that you can feel and see it with soft and moist skin.

Illnesses linked to lack of the lipids Omega 3 and vitamin D.

Medical problems related to a too low level of the essential fatty acid Omega 3 with DHA and EPA and the oil soluble vitamin D seems to be many. The list of illnesses where these lipids are involved seems also to increase each year with new research and understanding of their many functions in the body.

To get a brief overview of illnesses where the lack of Omega 3 and vitamin D are considered important I have collected general health information where these lipids were either listed as the main reason for the illness or a contributing reason or acted as a help to heal or relieve the illness. By digging deeper into the subject of illnesses and the healing of illnesses related to the lack of these lipids I am sure you will find more illnesses to add to the list. The difference between the Omega-3 and vitamin D in illnesses is difficult to evaluate so I have listed them together.

New research from some universities in the USA and Europe seems to conclude that you need up to 10 times the current daily recommendation of the oil soluble vitamin D to prevent some of the most serious illnesses we are facing today. This research comes at a time when a medical group involved in the setting of the daily recommendation state the current daily recommendation for the intake of vitamin D does not need major adjustments. It seems the current daily recommendation does not take into account all the new functions in the body where recent research has proven the oil soluble vitamin D is active, such as, regulating blood pressure, insulin production, regulation of the immune function and DNA and many other functions.

One doctor involved in a study of vitamin D since many years, now in a private organization with the name "Vitamin D Council", is of the opinion that we have a world-wide vitamin D deficiency of epidemic proportions with more than one billion people at risk for associated illnesses.

According to some doctor's vitamin D should not have been classified as a vitamin, as it acts more like a hormone in the body. The many functions of vitamin D are still not fully understood. What is understood is that vitamin D can heal and protect against illnesses.

Omega 3 with DHA and EPA and the oil soluble vitamin D seems to be listed as beneficial in the treatment or prevention of a number of illnesses as highlighted in the attached list, but please do not take the list as an extract from a medical research document. Instead, in case you are interested in some of the problems or illnesses listed do your own study. The purpose with the list of illnesses is to highlight there are a high number of illness where the lack of Omega 3 and vitamin D are considered important. The number of illnesses seems to increase each year, with a growing understanding of the many functions of the essential fatty acid Omega 3 and the oil soluble vitamin D:

1. Inflammation and inflammatory pain.
2. Arthritis and rheumatoid arthritis.
3. Bone and muscle pain and weakness.
4. Joint diseases and destruction of joint cartilage and rickets.
5. Hip fractures and osteoporosis.
6. Bleeding gums, inflammation in the gum and dental problems.
7. Tuberculosis, lung problems and pulmonary disorders.
8. Asthma.
9. Diabetes.

10. Kidney problems.
11. Heart problems.
12. High blood pressure/ hypertension.
13. Blood clumping help and thereby prevention of the formation of blood clots.
14. Blood circulation help. Protect arteries from build up of plaque.
15. Cholesterol and blood fat triglyceride reduction.
16. Irregular heartbeat help. Combat strokes.
17. Blood sugar improvement.
18. Varicose vein help.
19. PMS problem help.
20. Help against Endometriosis pain.
21. Important for partners planning to have children. Improves the chances of fertility. It seems lack of vitamin D can also be transferred to the child.
22. Prevent premature births, low birth weight and other birth complications.
23. Autism prevention and help.
24. Brain development in babies and children.
25. Depression and mood disorders improver.
26. Help against tiredness.
27. Brain & nervous system help.
28. Poor memory help.
29. Learning and behavioural problems in children.
30. Stress, anger, anxiety and fear modulator.
31. Macular degeneration and crusty dirt of the eye prevention.
32. Retina function of the eye improvements.
33. Hearing loss, ear noise and sounds in the ears. Tinnitus.
34. Digestive problems including ulcers.
35. Constipation and haemorrhoids.
36. Gout.
37. Skin disorders including Psoriasis.
38. Acne.
39. Heals dry skin and makes the skin soft and moist.
40. Help against oily skin.
41. Heals dry or cracked skin on the heels of the feet.

42. Help against wrinkles.
43. Brittle finger nails help.
44. Dry or brittle hair help.
45. Common cold prevention.
46. Chronic Fatigue Syndrome help.
47. Help against disturbances in the mucus membranes.
48. Improves the immune system i.e. considered as an immune system booster.
49. Cancer.
50. Parkinson, Multiple Sclerosis, Lupus and other autoimmune system illnesses support.

In the early years of the 1900, after the discovery of vitamin A, D and Omega 3, and before the blood tests for lipids were invented, doctors used the condition of the skin as an indication or barometer of the health condition of the person. Dry skin was considered as a normal indication of a dry body due to the lack of the important lipids. Dry skin was seen as a risk to obtain the associated illnesses. These days the list of associated illnesses is longer and seems to increase each year.

If you have reach the stage of some dry skin patches on your body you most likely have much more than dry skin on your body. You might have reached some dryness in all the approximately 100 trillions of cells throughout your body. All the cells in your body need lipids or lubrication i.e. your skin, your nails, your hair, your eyes, your ears, your joints, your bones, your digestion, your muscles, your nerves, your brain, your lungs, your hearth, your blood vessels and your blood cells etc, but you see and feel the lack of the important lipids best with your skin.

The skin is the organ in your body which gives up the important lipids first.

Dry skin or some of the other early warning signals give you a warning signal the cell membranes in all the trillions of cells in your body are in need of the lipids Omega 3 and vitamin A & D and the other lipids to function properly. Serious illnesses can take many years to reach a measureable level so it is important to correct dry skin and body as early as possible with the essential fatty acid Omega 3 and the oil soluble vitamin D plus the other oil soluble vitamins to start a healing process at the cellular level to prevent the development of illness.

Without proper lubrication the arteries are also slowly losing their elasticity and become hard and brittle, increasing the risk for possible hearth problems. Dry skin can also be an early warning signal the blood cells and blood plasma are slowly drying out and loosing the lubrication that allows the red blood cells to circulate freely into the smallest capillaries feeding each cell. The capillaries are the thin veins where only one blood cell at a time can pass through to bring oxygen, lipids and other nutrients to the cell.

According to the late Dr. M.H. Knisley/ USA, who was a recognized specialist on blood illnesses back in the 1940s, the red blood cells start to clump together and you get "sludging" or a clumping together of the red blood cells. According to Dr. Knisley, sludging or clumping of the red blood cells seems to be part of most degenerative illnesses or what is also named autoimmune system disorders these days with no real medical solution. According to the doctor cold hands and feet are early warning signs of sludged blood with bad blood circulation.

Dry skin patches can be the early warning signals before you reach the sludged blood situation!

Cancer is another illness where the lipids play a very import role and according to some reports natural occurring vitamin D is one of the most powerful cancer fighter ever discovered.

When the skin is dry there is a risk the essential oily coating which protects the nerves might lead to malfunctions of nerves causing many incurable nerve or muscle disorders. The brain depends on essential lipids for the proper mental function.

Rickets or softening of the bones was at a time a widespread illness related to lack of the oil soluble vitamin D. These days we have another widespread serious bone related illness with bone fractures and osteoporosis. Vitamin D plays an important role in the strength of the bones.

When the joints start to dry out you might end up with inflammatory arthritis which can be a painful inflammation reaction at the cellular level.

Inflammation is a healthy immune response to all kinds of infections, irritations, malfunctions and injury to the cells in the body. Short term inflammation is a normal immune system response to these reactions, but there are other types of inflammations which are not short term and they cause illness. Inflammation or oxidative stress at the cellular level is what many doctors believe is the start of most serious illnesses these days related to aging, heart, lung, cancer and many more.

Inflammation at the cellular level seems to start with malfunctions of the cell membranes due to lack of the important lipids in the cell membranes. When the cell membranes become dry due to lack of lipids the transport of nutrients into the cell through the cell membrane start to malfunction. Old nutrients or toxins leaving the cell face the same problem. With this cellular malfunction an inflammation or oxidative stress at the cellular level has started. With no healthy supply of the important lipids to improve the situation in the cell membranes the inflammation becomes permanent and illness will gradually develop over time.

With the supply of the natural essential fatty acid Omega 3 and the oil soluble vitamin D and the other lipids from the inside via the blood circulation, reaching all the trillions of cells, there is a good chance to prevent or reduce cellular inflammation. When the important lipids reach the cells the malfunction in the cell membranes can be healed or prevented. If inflammation has stated the inflammation should gradually be reduced and a healing process at the cellular level will start. Add pure water and alkaline food rich in trace minerals necessary for a healthy body and the cellular healing process will work even faster.

Why do you not hear more about the correct use of these important lipids which can prevent dry skin and body and can relive or cure so many illnesses, you might think or ask?

The newspapers, magazines and other news channels are full of information about food or supplements rich in Omega 3 and vitamin D, but does it work?

If the information regarding food and supplements had been correct and working the list of illness should be much shorter and not increasing!

Another issue to remember is the treatments with food or natural medicine are not really accepted by the medical community as medicine any longer, after we got our modern pharmaceutical industry in the 1950s. It does not matter if certain food and natural medicines have been used as medicine for hundreds of years. For this reason do not expect any help related to the use of old natural medicine from this professional group. The pharmaceutical industry with its powerful connections makes sure it stays that way.

The food suppliers or supplement suppliers are not able to guide you either except recommending you to eat food or take supplements rich in Omega 3 and vitamin D. From experience we know it does not work or we would have much less illnesses related to the lack of these important lipids.

When it comes to the use of natural medicines, natural medicines are no different than modern medicine. You need to know how to use natural medicine correctly to obtain the stated benefit. The information or guidance on the use of natural medicine is normally based on many years of use. The information has stayed in the families involved in the healing arts of herbs and natural medicines for many generations. The good thing with most natural medicines is that it contains no chemical toxins.

To guide us to obtain a healthy level of Omega 3 and vitamin D we can use the research and guideline discovered by the doctor in the USA who studied the illnesses of the metabolism and lipid metabolism with marine oil to obtain a healthy level of Omega 3 and vitamin A & D.

The good thing with his method to obtain Omega 3 and vitamin A & D and the other lipids the natural way is that you can both feel and see the progress with the lipid supplementation in your skin.

Water and oil or lipids do not mix or emulsify.

Contrary to most thinking, the body depends not only on what we eat and drink, but the most important part is probably the timing of the water or any other watery drink with the meal.

Without the correct timing of the water or any watery drink with the food very little of the important lipids Omega 3 and vitamin D in the food will reach and benefit the cells in the skin and body.

The doctor who studied illnesses of the metabolism and lipid metabolism with marine oil to obtain Omega 3 and vitamin A & D in the 1940s discovered water and oil or lipids do not mix or emulsify correctly in the digestive system. He discovered when food rich in oil or lipids was mixed with water or any other watery drink in the stomach during the meal the digestive process in the stomach would be affected in such a way that very little of the lipids in the oil or food rich in lipids would reach the cells in the skin. At that time the skin was used as a measuring point or barometer for the penetration of the lipids into the skin and body. By having the same meal without water, he discovered the lipids had no problem to reach the cells in the skin.

Oil and water do not mix or emulsify and it is easy to prove this at home. If we can accept this chemical condition the rest of his study becomes easier to understand.

The water or any other watery drink defined as an oil-free beverage, by the doctor, will interfere in the digestive processes of the food with oil or the lipids in such a way the oil or lipids will not be broken down correctly or emulsified correctly into the smallest building blocks with the rest of the food. Due to the incorrect emulsification process the lipids will be transferred wrongly into the body where most of the important lipids will remain in one organ, the liver. The liver, when we mix water and food with lipids, will only release small amounts of the healthy lipids into the blood circulation. The release is normally too small to heal or prevent the development of dry cells in the skin and body.

Our habit of drinking water or any other watery drink with food prevents a healthy level of the lipids in the food to reach the cells in the skin and body. This lack of the healthy lipids Omega 3 and vitamin D seems to be the main reason why we get dry skin and body and the many illnesses associated with a dry body.

The selection of food sources for our meals will also to a certain extent have an impact on the development of dry skin and body. Some food sources have less Omega 3 and vitamin A & D than other food sources. With the type of industrial farming we have these days some of the main food sources are having a low level of Omega 3 and vitamin D, and some food sources have too much of the wrong lipid Omega 6. Still the main reason for dry skin and body seems to be the wrong timing with the consumption of water or any other watery drink. The watery drink will prevent a natural break down or emulsification process with a correct absorption and transport of the major part of the healthy lipids into the cells of the skin and body.

For the major part of the important lipids in marine oil or food rich in these lipids to be able to reach the cells in your skin and body, you have to separate the food and water when you eat. You need to get into the very old habit used by our ancestors to drink your water when thirsty and 10 minutes or more before the food. This habit will enable the water to leave the stomach before the arrival of the food. No water or any other watery drink should now enter the stomach for 3 hours after the food. This will enable the digestion of the food to be completed correctly with a correct emulsification of the available lipids. This was all discovered by the doctor who studied the lipid metabolism with marine oil to obtain the important lipids Omega 3 and vitamin A & D into the cells of the skin and body.

With this habit or method of separating water and food the majority of the healthy lipids available in the food will always reach your cells in the skin and body.

This habit of drinking water when thirsty, before the food, was a natural habit of drinking water, most of the time, for a very large percentage of previous generations. They used this habit of drinking water most of their life, without even thinking about it.

They would normally drink their water when thirsty after waking up, walking, work, hunting, riding and cycling as most people had been doing for years before them.

Before the automobile, walking and cycling to and from work or shopping were normal. People became thirsty and they drank their water most of the time as soon as they came inside the door of their home to eat and rest to stop their thirst. Homemade soups were also used much more in the main meals those days than these days. Because of this natural way of drinking water when thirsty there was no need for them to drink more water during the meal, as they were not thirsty!

The natural food sources, with wild fish or free range animals with a natural diet and pesticide free fruit and berries and vegetables from chemical free soil, provided previous generations with food rich in the natural lipids of Omega 3 and vitamin A & D.

With all these natural food sources and natural habits of separating drinks and food previous generations received a much higher level of the essential fatty acids Omega 3 and the oil soluble vitamin D than most of us we can obtain today. With this healthy lipid protection they manage to avoid in a natural way a number of the most serious illnesses we are facing today.

How to bring a healthy level of the lipids Omega 3 and vitamin D into your cells?

The use of marine oils with Omega 3 and vitamin D and the other oil soluble vitamins to improve health seems to be easy to explain by doctors. However when we sit down to eat the food recommended to be rich in the healthy lipids something is happening to the lipids in the food or the supplements which cannot easily be explained, as we continue to get dry skin and body.

If you should take the time to ask old friends, friends who you know have been eating wild fish and taking marine oil supplementation most of their life, you will most likely discover that they have more or less the same problem as you might have, as their cells in the skin and body are also lacking the healthy lipids.

These days it seems to be normal for most people to have dry skin, hair and body when they reach a certain age. The unfortunate situation, which was discovered by doctors long time back, is that dry cells in the skin and body carries the risk of associated illnesses.

To obtain a healthy level of the lipids Omega 3 and vitamin D from food or supplements seems to be very difficult if not almost impossible for most of us these days. The reason for this problem is more or less the same today as it was for many people back in the early1900, when the doctors started to notice the development of various illnesses due to dry skin and body. The lipids and the water do not mix and emulsify. When we eat our food and drink our watery drinks the lipids in the food will not be emulsified correctly. For this reason the lipids will fail to find the correct transport channel to the cells in the skin and body.

If you should decide to test it out, as the doctor who studied the lipid metabolism with marine oils in the 1940s decided to do, you should be able to discover that the absorption of the lipids into the skin will depend very much if you drink water or any other watery drink with the food rich in lipids. You should also be able to discover that the temperature of the drink will have a very large impact on the lipid distribution to the cells in the skin and the body. With cold drinks you should be able to discover that hardly any of the healthy lipids reach the cells in the skin. If you should continue the test for some time, without drinking water during and after the meals, you should also be able to discover the high additional effect on the distribution of the lipids with the use of homemade soups and room tempered or warm whole milk. The use of homemade soups and room tempered or warm whole milk would give you an additional healthy level of the lipids to the cells in your skin and body. You would notice and feel it with your new soft and moist skin.

Why is there such a big difference in the lipid distribution to the cells of the skin and the body when the food ingredients in the meals are basically the same? The only difference is the water. The watery drink interferes in the chemical process which takes place in your stomach when you eat food with lipids.

The entry of water or any other watery drink into the digestive process with the lipids is the main reason to the problem of not receiving a healthy level of Omega 3 and vitamin D into the cells of the skin and body. This problem was discovered by the doctor who studied the lipid metabolism with marine oils to obtain a healthy level of the important lipids Omega 3 and vitamin A & D into the cells of the skin.

Water and oil or lipids do not mix or emulsify. The water or any other watery drink which enter the stomach with the food will interfere in the digestive process of the food. The digestive process is a kind of chemical process. For whatever reason the molecular end product of the food, after the chemical digestive process or break down process to the smallest building blocks or molecules, is different with water compared to no water. The same happens to the molecular end products when we eat homemade soups or room tempered whole milk with the food, without water, but now almost all the lipid molecular end products manage to reach the cells in the skin and body.

After the digestion when the lipid molecular end products together with all the other molecular end products from the food start their journey into the digestive pipe or intestine pipe to be absorbed into the transport channel to feed the cells in the skin and body something will cause that much less of the important lipids reach the cells in the skin and body when there is water mixed into the molecular end products. With water or any other watery drink the important lipids in the food seems not to be able to leave the liver to reach the cells in the skin and body at a healthy level. For this reason we get dry skin and body over time. By eating the same type of marine oil or food rich in lipids, but without drinking water or any other watery drink during the digestive process of the lipids much more of the healthy lipids reach the cells in the skin and body.

To repeat what the doctor discovered with his study of the lipid metabolism: Drink your water or any watery drink 10 minutes before the food and have no water or any watery drink during the digestive period for up to 3 hours after the food.

The importance with a separation of water and food to assist the digestion has also been confirmed by other doctors before the discovery the lipids and water do not mix or emulsify and now more recently by another doctor who studied water and health in the USA.

As far as I know there has not been published any research on the lipid metabolism with marine oils known to be rich in the important essential fatty acid Omega 3 and the oil soluble vitamin D since the study made by the doctor in the 1940s. For whatever reason, it seems his research on the lipid metabolism with marine oil to obtain a healthy level of Omega 3 and vitamin A & D to prevent dry skin and body and the associated illnesses was considered unimportant by the medical establishment at that time.

New research in the field of the healthy lipids seems to be focused mostly on finding and treating illnesses related to the lack of Omega 3 and vitamin D with chemical medicine instead of trying to find out how to heal and prevent illness the natural way with Omega 3 and vitamin D from food or supplements.

With this brief overview of the study on the lipid metabolism with marine oils to bring a healthy level of Omega 3 and vitamin D and the other lipids and the explanations of the many changes which have affected our habits or ability to obtain a healthy level of the lipids Omega 3 and vitamin D to heal and prevent dry skin and body your question might be:

How can we use the doctor's research to obtain the important essential fatty acid Omega 3 with DHA and EPA and the oil soluble vitamin D and the other lipids into our cells in our skin and body to avoid dry skin and body and the many associated illnesses?

We would like to continue to have our various drinks with our meals as these drinks have become an important part or habit of our life.

We do not have time to search for wild fish, free-range eggs and chicken and grass feed beef, fruit, berries and vegetables from chemical free soil or other food sources known to be rich in the healthy lipids Omega 3 and vitamin D.

We have hardly any time to prepare and eat homemade soups and we might even like to continue to use tinned or canned food, even if the study of the doctor indicate that we would hardly get any of the important lipids from such food.

We might however try to be more out in the sun, but . . . .

To understand what we need to do to obtain a healthy level of the lipids Omega 3 and vitamin D from the food, with the above mentioned wish list or objection to change, we need to use the research on lipid metabolism made by the doctor and let his research guide us. Based on his research, there seems to be only two methods to bring a healthy level of the essential fatty acid Omega 3 and the oil soluble vitamin D together with the other lipids into the cells in the skin and body, and I will name them, the original method and the modern method.

The original method has been used by our ancestors for thousands of years. They had a natural habit of drinking water when thirsty. With this habit most of them managed to separate water and food in most of their meals and in this way they managed to obtain a healthy level of the lipids. I will not repeat this method, but if you decide to follow this original method it should work over time. Find natural food rich in the healthy lipids and use the old cooking methods with homemade soups or stew. Some natural exposure to the sun should also help.

The modern method is a method which is much more suitable to our existing lifestyle and habit with food and water together in our meals. With this habit of drinking any watery drink during your meal you can basically forget to get a healthy level of the healthy lipids Omega 3 and vitamin D from food or supplements rich in these lipids. The watery drink during the digestive process will prevent it.

Instead, if you have a wish to obtain a healthy level of Omega 3 and vitamin D, you need to take Omega 3 and vitamin D separately from any food and watery drink. For this reason the modern method is based on a supplementation method with marine oil. The supplementation method will follow the process or method the doctor discovered with his research on lipid metabolism with a small refinement introduced by another health focused person to make it more adoptable to our modern life. The marine oil will be emulsified to help to release the lipids in the marine oil. The emulsification process will also change the taste of the marine oil.

The modern method with supplementation with marine oil, the correct way, with an emulsification process will allow you much more freedom in your habits of food and drinks, but even this modern method to obtain the healthy level of Omega 3 and vitamin D, will not be able to bypass the old discovery that oil or lipids do not mix with water or any other watery drink or what was defined as an oil-free beverage. For this reason there will still be some small restrictions, regarding the use of water or any other watery drink before and after the use of this modern method to obtain a healthy level of Omega 3 and vitamin D.

The modern method with a supplementation with emulsified marine oil is probably the best and only method available today to obtain a healthy level of Omega 3 and the oil soluble vitamin D and the other lipids from marine oil supplements rich in these important lipids. The good thing with this method to obtain a healthy level of the important lipids is that you can feel and see it with moist and soft skin after a couple of months. Gradually over time after the trillions of cells in the body fills up with the healthy lipids other more important health benefits might be felt.

What type of marine oil to use as a supplement, fish or Cod liver oil?

Marine oils or Cod liver oils with their special healing power were researched extensively by Dr. Ludovicus J. de Jongh from Holland in the period 1840s to 1860s. Dr. de Jongh published his first medical report in 1842 covering different illnesses which he had treated successfully over a period of more than 10 years with the use of Cod liver oil. The year after, in 1843, Dr. de Jongh published his first chemical analysis of Cod liver oil. Dr. John Bennett from Scotland reported in 1841 his medical observations with the use of Cod liver oil as medicine from his visit to Germany, where he had observed treatments for bone illnesses and other illnesses with the use of Cod liver oil.

Before these official medical publications on the use of Cod liver oil to treat various illnesses, doctors and people living in the fishing communities bordering the cold North Sea with Norway, Denmark, Germany, Holland, Scotland and England had discovered and used the health benefit of raw Cod liver oil for many years for the healing of deformed bones, rickets, rheumatism, aches, pain and other illnesses.

According to old import recordings discovered in German and English ports, Cod liver oil has been imported from Bergen in Norway by these two countries for more than 800 years. From Dr. J. Bennett's medical report we know the German doctors used Cod liver oil as medicine to heal various illnesses before the year 1841. As Cod liver oil was also used for other purposes than medicine there are no recordings which year Cod liver oil was first used as medicine, but it should be safe to assume it started much earlier than 1841.

Dr. de Jongh concluded already in 1846 there were different types or qualities of Cod liver oil available in the fish market. He discovered first the difference in the quality with the Cod liver oils with the healing results he obtained with his patients. From the fish market he got different types of Cod liver oils. Through his medical research and chemical analysis of the Cod liver oils he was able to select the Cod liver oil with the best healing result for his patients. He discovered some of the merchants dealing in fish and marine oils used to mix fish oils with Cod liver oils. When the merchants mixed fish oils with the Cod liver oil, Dr. de Jongh discovered he got Cod liver oil which had much less healing power for his patients.

The only long term medical evaluation of the healing power of fish oil and Cod liver oil on health and different illnesses seems to be the approximately 10 years medical study published by Dr. de Jongh in 1842. With his chemical analysis of Cod liver oil in 1843 and his medical study of his patients over many years Dr. de Jongh concluded already in 1846 that fish oil did not have the medical healing power of quality Cod liver oil.

Dr. de Jongh, based on his medical studies and chemical analysis, concluded the only Cod liver oil to be used as medicine was the light brown Cod liver oil extracted from the cod fish living in cold arctic waters.

There have also been more recent evaluations of marine oils and other healthy oils by people with long experience of studying the health aspect of oils. From what I understand, they never really managed to find out the reason why Cod liver oil was superior to other oils in the healing process of the cells in the skin and body. One person who studied the healing power of Cod liver oil and other healthy oils in the skin and body for more than 40 years concluded, as Dr. de Jongh did in 1846, the health benefit of Cod liver oil from the cod fish living in the arctic sea is special. He concluded the special healing power of Cod liver oil must come from the many ingredients only available in the diet to the cod fish in the cold arctic sea waters.

It has been known for a very long time the liver of any animal contains the highest quality of nutritional reserves of the whole body. When we use Cod liver oil from the Cod fish from the cold arctic sea we are getting a concentrate of the best nutrition the arctic sea can provide.

What type of Cod liver oil to use?

The only long term medical evaluation of Cod liver oil as medicine for different illnesses seems to be the medical publication published by Dr. de Jongh in 1842 and his chemical analysis of Cod liver oil published in 1843.

Dr. de Jongh concluded based on his long medical research with his patients and chemical analysis of different Cod liver oils he obtained the best medical healing power with the Cod liver oil from the cod fish living in the cold arctic water off the coast of Norway.

With his chemical analysis of Cod liver oil, which was first performed in 1843, before the discovery of the oil soluble vitamins and the essential fatty acids in Cod liver oil in the early years of the 1900, Dr. de Jongh managed to identify 17 different acids and trace minerals including Iodine and some fatty acids. The fatty acids were later in the 1930s discovered and named the essential fatty acid Omega 3 and Omega 6.

Dr. de Jongh used Cod liver oil successfully as medicine for many different illnesses for many years. To ensure he would be able to get the best Cod liver oil for his medical practice he decided to visit the Norwegian producer of Cod liver oil in 1846.

With the medical success Dr. de Jongh received, he decided in 1850, to make the high quality Cod liver oil from Norway available as a medicine to a much larger population. His Cod liver oil bearing the name "Dr. de Jongh's Light Brown Cod Liver Oil" was marketed throughout Europe and USA. Each bottle carried a Dr. de Jongh seal guaranteeing the product had passed a chemical analysis.

More recently, other people who have been studying fish and marine oils are of the same opinion as Dr. de Jongh, the fish to be able to produce any good lipids Omega 3 with DHA and EPA and the oil soluble vitamin D, needs to live in cold waters to obtain a diet producing the important lipids.

The discoveries made by Dr. de Jongh and others more recently should also be considered when you buy and eat fish to obtain the essential fatty acid Omega 3 and vitamin D. Most fish these days might come from a fish farm where the diet available to the fish will limit the production of the important lipids in the fish. The fish might look the same and have tasty protein fish meat, but most likely there are very little of the important essential fatty acid Omega 3 with DHA and EPA and the oil soluble vitamin D in the fish.

Resent research on fish oils conclude also there is a difference in the nutritional values between fish oils from wild fish and fish oil from farmed fish.

Due to the importance of the diet for the fish to produce Omega 3 and vitamin D, the Cod liver oil extracted from the cod fish from the cold arctic waters off the coast of North of Norway seems still to be best source of Cod liver oil. This type of Cod liver oil is also normally guaranteed free from mercury and other toxins and has vitamin E added from a natural source to keep it fresh for a long period of time.

Different Norwegian Cod liver oil manufacturers exist, but the best Norwegian Cod liver oil seems to be the Cod liver oil manufactured by the old Cod liver oil company "Peter Moller". Peter Moller established their present Cod liver oil business in Norway in 1854, based on an existing Cod liver oil business.

Outside Norway I understand "Carlson Norwegian" Cod liver oil is rated the best Cod liver oil. The "Carlson Norwegian" Cod liver oil is supplied by "Peter Moller" in Norway and carries the same guaranty of potency and purity as the original Peter Moller Cod liver oil product sold in Norway under the old Norwegian name "Tran".

The "Peter Moller" Cod liver oil which is called "Tran" in Norway and the "Carlson Norwegian" Cod liver oil in liquid form are available in two flavours, natural flavour or lemon flavour. Both flavours will give the same result in your skin and body, so it is only a preference of flavour when selecting the Cod liver oil, from these suppliers. Most people select the lemon flavour.

If you are afraid of the fishy flavour from the Cod liver oil, relax. To obtain a maximum healthy benefit from the Cod liver oil you will have to mix it with something, which will be explained later, which will turn it into a more pleasant drink. For this reason the Cod liver has to be liquid.

The "Carlson Norwegian" Cod liver oil contains approximately the following oil soluble vitamins and the essential fatty acids per table spoon of 5ml:

Omega 3 Fatty Acid,	1,100mg
DHA	500mg
EPA	400mg
ALA	40mg
Vitamin D	400IU
Vitamin A	850IU
Vitamin E	10IU

The Peter Moller, "Tran", sold in Norway, has slightly improved values for DHA and vitamin D. The products are guaranteed free of mercury, lead and other contaminants. The Cod liver oil is separated from the liver tissue from fresh cod fish found in the arctic water outside the coast of Norway.

Vitamin A and vitamin D, both natural parts of the Cod liver oil cooperate with one another in a natural way in the Cod liver oil. Old medical studies have found the vitamin D needs the help of vitamin A to work effectively in the body.

Other healthy ingredients in the Cod liver oil from the arctic sea water are not declared, by the supplier. The ocean water since millions of years contains more than 70 different trace minerals including Iodine originally washed into the sea from the mountains and soil. These trace minerals are identified in sea salts. With these trace minerals part of the sea water there is a good chance that a healthy level of many of these important trace minerals are part of the nutrients stored in the liver of the cod fish and are part of the Cod liver oil.

I have used Cod liver oil before and I did not notice any difference in my skin.

Many people might say that they have already tried and used Cod liver oil before, but they did not notice any difference in the skin or body as the use of Cod liver oil with Omega 3 and vitamin D is nothing new.

Until some time ago I belonged to that group too, but I am now a devoted emulsified Cod liver oil fan. The same is my wife and some friends. The emulsified method of taking the Cod liver oil does work. It gives you results which you can both see and feel in your skin with a gradual improvement with soft moist skin within a period of approx. 1 1/2 to 3 months. The complete treatment to obtain soft and moist skin takes longer and it depends on the dryness in the trillions of cells of your skin and body.

The reason for previous lack of healing response with the use of Cod liver oil, if you have used it before, could have been some of the following reasons:

- Did not emulsify the Cod liver oil before taking it.
- Drank water or other watery drink just before the Cod liver oil.
- Drank water or other watery drink when taking the Cod liver oil.
- Drank water or other watery drink within the digestive period after taking the Cod liver oil.
- Took Cod liver oil as capsules.

- Eat food, medicine, fruits or other ingredients in the stomach before taking the Cod liver oil.
- Eat food, medicine, fruits or other ingredients after taking the Cod liver oil.
- Other influences on the digestive process immediately before or after taking the Cod liver oil.

I can still remember my childhood years in Norway, in the 1950s, when we had to take Cod liver oil by the spoon. At that time you had to take it as it was supposed to be good for you. That was the message from my mother. Hardly any person questioned what good the Cod liver oil would do as it was recommended to be good for the children and pregnant women by the Health Authority.

I can still remember that it tasted bad. These days you can at least get Cod liver oil with lemon flavour. The emulsification process described and proposed, which is required to obtain a healthy level of the important lipids from the Cod liver oil, will also improve the flavour of the oil.

From what I understand many people still take their Cod liver oil, by the tea or table spoon or capsules, but I must admit that I have not met people so far who have notice a real difference in their skin or body when taking it. Surely it must do something good for someone as Cod liver oil has been used for a long time, but until recently I have failed to discover the real healing power of Cod liver oil.

As explained earlier, a large percentage of previous generations, due to their work and living conditions and habits would most likely have consumed their water before the meals. Most likely they followed the water separately when they had their Cod liver oil as medicine. Due to the strong flavour of the Cod liver oil at that time they might even have emulsified it, without knowing the effect of it, by eating a warm homemade soup afterwards to remove the flavour of the Cod liver oil or mixing it into the soup. As far as I can remember from my child hood days in Norway, we used milk and food to remove the flavour of the oil, but our food was not compatible with the food which would give a high percentage of the lipids Omega 3 and vitamin A & D into the cells of the skin and body. In other words, my parents did not know how to use the natural medicine of Cod liver oil correctly to obtain a high healthy level of the important Omega 3 and vitamin A & D from it and neither did the Health Authority who recommended people to use the Cod liver oil.

Personally I thought for a long time, the Cod liver oil you get today and even back in my childhood days was different from the Cod liver oil used in the old days. I thought the Cod liver oil in the old days was mostly raw or fermented. The Cod liver oil we got as children and what we can buy today is heat treated in a special method to eliminate impurities and improve the taste and storage time. I thought the heat treatment, made the oil to loose most if not all of its health benefits. Only recently did I discover the special heat treatment method was invented in Norway already in the early 1860's or even earlier by the Peter Moller company and has been used, with various additional improvements over the years, since the 1860s.

I must admit I still have some problems to understand the heat treatment method used to clean, flavour and improve the storage time of the Cod liver oil, does not remove some of the health benefits in the natural Cod liver oil. Whatever natural lipids of Omega 3 with DHA and EPA and vitamin A and D and other lipids and trace minerals which are left in the Cod liver oil after the treatment there must be sufficient to do a lot of good in the cells of the skin and body, as my dry skin disappeared after less than 2 months after I started to take the emulsified Cod liver oil according to the correct emulsification method.

It took me more than 10 years to come to this conclusion. I got the first information on the emulsification process of the Cod liver oil from a friendly health "guru" long time back. He recommended me to obtain the book and try it for my digestive problems, at that time. When I discovered the Cod liver oil recommended to be used was still the same type of heat treated Cod liver oil I was used to from my childhood days in Norway, I decide it was not worth the test and I filed the Cod liver oil document in my filing system.

Due to my fixed idea the Cod liver oil had to be raw and unheated to protect the living enzymes in the oil, to give real valuable health contribution, I did not study Cod liver oil further. As I understood Omega 3 and other lipids were important for health I continued to eat good food as most people. I also continued to read and collect whatever new and old information I could get hold off related to Cod liver oil, Omega 3 and vitamin D and other healthy oils for many years. My reading and collection of information on Cod liver oil and other healthy oils continued at this level for more than 10 years until one day in 2010, I decided to have a second look at the old Cod liver oil document, I had filed. This time, after more than 10 years of study of many health documents, the emulsification process of the Cod liver oil described sounded interesting. I could now see and understand the similarities with an emulsification method discovered by Dr. Johanna Budwig, a German doctor, with her flax seed oil or linseed oil mixed or rather emulsified in low fat quark or cottage cheese which is a sulphur rich protein. By this time I had already tested out the Dr. J. Budwig flaxseed oil and quark mixture for more than 2 years, with good detoxification results, but with no improvements for my dry skin. As I now had reached the level of very dry skin on my legs and other parts, and the emulsified Cod liver oil promised healing of dry skin within a relative short period of time I thought it would be easy to test it out.

You can probably imagine my surprise when I noticed a positive difference in my dry skin condition after approx. 1 ½ month. I noticed it first on my hands when washing as the water appeared as small droplets on my skin after washing. As I do not use any cream or oil to soften my skin, I was very surprised.

The next discovery came approximately 1 month later. This time I noticed the dryness or flakiness of the skin on my legs had vanished and the skin on my legs appeared moist. No more dryness or flakiness on the skin of my legs! The skin on the legs appeared moist after less than 3 months daily consumption of emulsified Cod liver oil, the correct way.

As we live in a warm climate with lots of sunshine I spend some time out in the sun at the swimming pool or sea during the week-ends, without applying any sun-cream, so my thoughts have always been that this exposure to the sun without a sun cream must be the main reason for my dry skin, but now I know the real reason. The cells in my skin and the body were drying out from the inside due to lack of the essential fatty acids Omega 3 and the oil soluble vitamin A and D.

My more or less weekly sun exposure to get a nice tan and my healthy and mostly organic food rich in Omega 3 and vitamin D did not help me much as I was drinking water, espresso or other watery drinks with my meals. These drinks disturbed the digestive process of the important lipids Omega 3 and the oil soluble vitamin D in the food.

The mixing of my food and watery drinks worked exactly as the doctor in the USA had discovered in his research on the marine oil metabolism. The watery drinks with the food prevented the important lipids Omega 3 and the oil soluble vitamin A and D in my food to be digested and emulsified correctly to enable the lipids to enter the correct transport channel into the circulating blood to reach the cells of my skin. With my habit of always drinking watery drinks with the food, only a small percentage of the available lipids in my food, rich in the important lipids, reached the cells of my skin. This small level of the available lipids was not sufficient to prevent me from getting very dry skin and body.

The days I enjoyed a cold drink with my fish meals the cells in my skin and body received hardly any of the healthy Omega 3 and vitamin A & D available in the fish.

My skin was the real proof of it with constant and increasing dryness.

My skin was drying out from the inside out, like the rest of my body. My good food and more or less weekly sun exposure most of the year without sun protection could not prevent it. Perhaps I shall also add that I used to drink fresh carrot juice made with a high quality hydraulic press juicer, each day for the last 12 years and this daily injection of fresh vegetable juice with lots of important nutrients did not help my cells in my skin and body from drying out either. The fresh daily carrot juice probably helped my body in many other areas, but my cells were still lacking the important lipids and they were drying out!

My experience with the emulsified Cod liver oil mixture, the correct way, was unbelievable.

My skin turned from dry to moist over a few months and other people are having the same experience with their dry skin or dry cells in the skin.

By taking the emulsified Cod liver oil mixture on an empty stomach with no food, fruit, snacks, water, medicines or any other items for 1 hour afterwards I do not need to think about my dry skin and body anymore. My skin on my hands and legs are now soft and moist without applying any cream or lotions. I can now also feel the lipids in the Cod liver oil have started to do other good things in my body.

After approx. 4-5 months after I started taking the emulsified Cod liver oil, I started to notice some changes in the cracking sounds in the bones when doing my various bending exercises. I have been doing these exercises regularly for more than 15 years with my old bones so I am very familiar with the old bone sounds, but now it feels that something is cushioning the sound.

The dry and thick skin on the heels and under the sole of my feet has also almost completely disappeared. It has been replaced with soft new skin after approximately 7 months on the emulsified Cod liver oil mixture. I noticed it first when walking on the hot stone surface at the swimming pool. Previously with my thick skin sole I could easily walk barefoot on the hot stone surface. Not anymore, with my thin and soft skin under the sole.

After approximately 8-9 months on the emulsified Cod liver oil mixture I discovered when cleaning my ears with Q-tips the return of some of the important yellow earwax.

I am still taking the emulsified Cod liver oil mixture daily in the morning on an empty stomach with no food or water for one hour afterwards as I still feel the emulsified Cod liver oil improves my bones and digestion.

When you start to correct dry skin and body the largest organ, the skin will correct first and then gradually the other organs and parts of the body will receive a higher percentage of the available lipids with each new supply.

The fact that many people have all forms of dry skin or other health conditions, even at a young age, should also indicate that the lipid distribution or absorption into the cells in body is mostly going wrong during the digestion. This is perhaps not so strange with all the new soft drinks, sport drinks and coffee drinks and other drinks which are consumed on a regular basis with snacks or food these days.

With the research on the lipid metabolism with marine oils performed by the doctor in the USA, I can now understand why most people do not see or feel any real result by taking their Cod liver oil supplements or eating fat wild fish or grass feed beef, free-range eggs or other food rich in these important lipids and I hope you have somehow reached the same understanding.

The water or any other watery drink with the food interrupt the digestion of the oily lipid molecules in the food so there will be a chemical process preventing a correct emulsification of the lipids in the digestive system which will cause the majority of the lipids to end up in the wrong transport channel into the body where it will do no good for the cells in the skin and body to improve health.

We need many more nutrients than the essential fatty acid Omega 3 and the oil soluble vitamin A and D so I will continue to eat healthy food, both with and without watery drinks.

One good thing with the emulsified Cod liver oil supplement method is that I can now always manage to supply my skin and body with a healthy level of the essential fatty acid Omega 3 with DHA and EPA and the oil soluble vitamin A and D + E as all these important lipids are normally included as natural lipids in a bottle of Cod liver oil of good quality.

The other good thing with the emulsified Cod liver oil supplement method is that I can easily see and feel the penetration level of the important lipids Omega 3 and vitamin A & D into the cells of my skin and body by checking the moisture of the skin on my legs and using the Q-tips in my ears.

It is that simple!

How do you obtain Omega 3 and vitamin D from Cod liver oil?

You can obtain the essential fatty acid Omega 3 and the oil soluble vitamin D and the other oil soluble vitamins from Cod liver oil, but to obtain a healthy level of the important lipids to prevent dry cells of the skin, hair and body you need to emulsify or mix the Cod liver oil with another liquid. There are also other certain important conditions you have to follow. The Cod liver oil has to be liquid and not in capsule form. It was all discovered by the doctor who studied illnesses of the metabolism and lipid metabolism with marine oil or Cod liver oil in the 1940s and another person who in the 1950s discovered and improved his discovery:

1. To obtain the maximum healthy benefit from the lipids Omega 3 and vitamin D and the other lipids in Cod liver oil you have to mix or emulsify the Cod liver oil with another liquid. You drink the emulsified Cod liver oil mixture on an empty stomach. An empty stomach means no food, snacks, medicines, coffee, tea or other items for 4 hours before taking the emulsified Cod liver oil mixture.
2. After you have taken the Cod liver oil mixture you have to keep a waiting period of 1 hour. During this waiting period you are not allowed to drink water or any other watery drink, or to eat food, snacks, medicines, or fruits or any other ingredients.
3. The drink has to be at room temperature when you drink it.

NOTE: If you are worried about the flavour of the drink the additional liquid will also improve the flavour of the drink.

That's it.

By following this special method of taking the Cod liver oil drink your dry cells will obtain a healthy level of Omega 3 and vitamin D and the other lipids from the emulsified Cod liver oil drink. The good thing with this method to obtain a healthy level of the lipids Omega 3 and vitamin D is that you can monitor the healing process with your skin. The lipids in the drink will start a healing process in the cells in the body at the cellular level. The skin is the organ which will receive the lipids first. The other organs and the rest of the body will follow. You should be able to see and feel a difference in your skin within 1-3 months depending on the dryness of your skin and body when you started.

With this method of taking the Cod liver oil you can still continue with your existing habit of having a watery drink with your meals, as long as you can find the correct time to take the emulsified Cod liver oil drink with the conditions as described above.

I believe most people who used to take Cod liver oil in the old days had a natural habit to separate water and food. They probably also used an emulsification process to get it down, due to the awful flavour of the Cod liver oil at that time. I would not be surprised if the emulsification process would be a warm soup or stew without water or any other watery drink, as explained earlier. In this way the people would automatically get up to 10 times or even close to 20 times the lipids you would get by eating a wild fat salmon fish or similar fish with a cold drink, these days.

How do you emulsify the Cod liver oil?

The Cod liver oil is emulsified or mixed by shaking it with an oil bearing liquid. Whole milk or normal full fat milk is an oil bearing liquid and this milk is used to emulsify the Cod liver oil.

The emulsification process, with mixing the two liquids is performed by shaking the liquids in a small screw top glass jar. The emulsification or mixing shall be performed just before you drink the emulsified Cod liver oil and milk drink. The mixture shall be kept at room temperature when you emulsify and drink it. For this reason prepare the milk and Cod liver oil mixture according to the description below, in advance, and leave it outside the fridge until you decide to emulsify and drink it.

For the best time to drink the emulsified Cod liver oil, to obtain a healthy level of Omega 3 and vitamin A & D into the cells of the skin and body from the drink, see the description below.

To start you need the following:
Tools:
1. One clean screw top glass jar with a good screw cap. The glass jar should take approximately 6 fluid ounces of liquid or the equivalent to 1, 5 decilitres of liquid. For selection of screw top glass jars see more information at the bottom of next page.
2. Table spoon or tea spoon to be used for measurement.
3. Watch with indicator for seconds, to take the time while shaking the glass jar.

Ingredients:
4. Whole milk, approximately 9 table spoons or 2 fluid ounces or 50ml or ½ decilitre.
5. Cod liver oil, 1 table spoon or 1 tea spoon, depending on the age as outlined below.

Start by selecting a screw top glass jar with size as described above. Pour the whole milk, with approximately 9 full table spoons, into the screw top glass jar and add a full table spoon with Cod liver oil to the milk for an adult. The total volume with 9+1=10 tablespoons should fill approximately 1/3 of the screw top glass jar with size as described above. For new born babies up to the age of 6 months reduce the Cod liver oil to 1 tea spoon, but keep the milk the same.

The measurement and procedure can also be explained as follows:
Pour approximately 2 fluid ounces of whole milk with one table spoon of cod liver oil into the screw top glass jar. Two fluid ounces of whole milk is the equivalent to approximately 50ml or ½ decilitre.

After you have filled the milk and the Cod liver oil inside the screw top glass jar you should have approximately 2/3 of empty space inside the glass jar to be used for the emulsification or shaking process. The screw top glass jar should not have too much empty space inside or too much of the liquid will cling to the surface of the glass jar and be lost during the emulsification or shaking process. This is the reason for the selected size of the screw top glass jar. After you have filled the whole milk and the Cod liver oil inside the glass jar you should make sure that the screw cap or lid for the glass jar is secure and completely tight. To simplify the work with the milk pouring try to remember the level of milk in the glass jar or mark the glass jar with a permanent marker pen. The volume of milk is approximately so a little more or a little less milk make no difference.

To emulsify the Cod liver oil and milk you need to shake the glass jar vigorously for approx. 15 seconds, but not before you decide to drink it.

The milk should not be cold, but the milk should have room temperature so plan accordingly. Leave the drink outside the fridge over night after pouring it, if you plan to take it during the night or in the morning. Should you forget to take the milk and the Cod liver oil out of the fridge so the drink is cold, heat the glass jar with the drink inside in warm water for a few minutes. This should enable it to reach room temperature.

To emulsify the drink shake the screw top glass jar for 15 seconds. Take the time on your watch, until you can manage to guess the approximate time. Drink the emulsified Cod liver oil and milk mixture immediately, preferably from the glass jar to obtain as much as possible of the content.

NOTE: You need to drink it on an empty stomach, and you are not allowed to drink, eat or take any medicine, snacks or drinks for 1 hour after the drink.

An empty stomach means no food, snacks, medicine, or complex drinks such as coffee, tea or other drinks for 4 hours before you take the emulsified Cod liver oil. The only exception to this rule is room tempered or warm water or whole milk. If you drink some room tempered or warm water or whole milk before the emulsified Cod liver oil drink, remember to wait a minimum of 10-15 minutes, before you emulsify the Cod liver oil and drink it. Do not drink any cold water or milk drink before the emulsified Cod liver oil drink as the cold drinks will affect the absorption rate of the emulsified Cod liver oil drink.

Do not make any changes to the above rule of taking the emulsified Cod liver oil, or the absorption rate and result will be reduced. Even a small content such as a capsule of Cod liver oil will interfere in the absorption rate of the Cod liver oil and this is the reason for the use of liquid or bottled Cod liver oil.

Another good thing with the emulsified Cod liver oil and milk drink is that the strong Cod liver oil flavour is disappearing and the drink now look and taste almost as a normal mini milk shake. Personally I think even a child will willingly take it and probably even ask for it if you explain what it can do for the child related to skin beauty and health.

If you decide to take the emulsified Cod liver oil drink in the early morning, it is recommended that you pour the milk and the Cod liver oil into the screw top glass jar in the evening and leave the glass jar outside the fridge to take it at room temperature the next morning.

For more detailed information and guidelines on how to find the best time to take the emulsified Cod liver oil drink, please refer to chapter **"When is the best time to take the emulsified Cod liver oil?"**

As the screw top glass jars can leak you should preferably do the shaking of the glass jar in the kitchen water area or bathroom without lifting it too high in the air in case the screw cap is not fully tight. To avoid a leak from the screw cap, when you shake the glass jar, it is recommended to press down the screw cap with the use of the thumb finger.

To obtain good screw top glass jars, in case you do not have them already in-house, buy some small English mustard screw top glass jars or similar screw top glass jars with net weight content of approximately 180-250 grams. The screw cap on these glass jars are designed to seal the glass jar after several open-close operations. Clean and wash them out in very hot water. Should it be difficult to remove the glue on the glass jar after the label has been removed you can remove the glue easily with a little spirit or lighter fuel on a paper towel. It is recommended to buy more than one glass jar per person so that you do not need to clean the glass jar immediately after use. It is best to buy only one make of jars to avoid leaks and mixing up the different sizes of caps. When one screw cap is worn out replace the entire set of jars to avoid mixing the screw caps.

What type of milk to use for the emulsification process?

Only normal whole milk can be used for the process of emulsification of the Cod liver oil to obtain the desired effect i.e. no low fat, skimmed or powder milk.

Whole milk, contains approx. 87% water, but it is still an oil bearing liquid. This is the reason that whole milk is able to emulsify Cod liver oil, under the previous specified conditions.

The milk to be used should be at room temperature when you plan to emulsify and drink it. For this reason if you store the milk in the fridge get into the habit of pouring the milk and the Cod liver oil into the screw top glass jar a few hours before you plan to use it or preferably the night before you plan to emulsify and drink it. The whole milk and the Cod liver oil can sit in the glass jar outside the fridge for many hours in normal room temperature without being spoilt.

What do you do if you are allergic to milk?

If you are allergic to milk, it is possible to use the same amount of fresh orange juice. The orange juice has to be made from fresh oranges. The juice has to be completely free from any fruit pulp and fruit fibres as this pulp and fruit fibre content will influence the digestive process. For this reason it will be necessary to strain the fresh orange juice directly after the juicing through a fine tea filter or fabric, to remove the pulp.

One normal size orange has normally approximately 9 to 11 table spoons of orange juice. The method with pulp free fresh orange juice emulsified with the Cod liver oil is not as effective as Cod liver oil with whole milk so expect that this method will take more time.

I personally have not tried it out, so I cannot give you a time table for the results, but as a worst case scenario expect a month or perhaps two months more to obtain a visible result in your skin and hair than using the emulsified Cod liver and milk method.

According to the doctor who discovered the emulsification process with the Cod liver oil, the emulsification process with room tempered orange juice will work, and the good thing with both the whole milk emulsification method and the orange juice emulsification method is that you should be able to see and feel the improvements in your skin and hair after a few months with a daily intake of the emulsified drink.

When is the best time to take the emulsified Cod liver oil?

To obtain a high and healthy level of the essential fatty acid Omega 3 and vitamin A & D from the Cod liver oil into the cells of the skin, hair and body there are some very important guidelines or rules which have to be followed:

Guideline 1 or Rule 1. It is necessary to take the emulsified Cod liver with milk on an empty stomach. An empty stomach means no food, snacks, medicines or complex drinks for approximately 4 hours.

Guideline 2 or Rule 2. After you have taken the emulsified Cod liver oil with milk you have a waiting period of 1 hour. During this 1 hour waiting period no food, medicine, snack, drink or anything else is allowed into the stomach. It is very important that nothing interfere in the digestion of the emulsified Cod liver oil and milk during this waiting period. Nothing!

Regarding drinks, you can drink room tempered water or warm water 10-12 minutes before you take your emulsified Cod liver oil and milk drink. The room tempered or warm water takes approximately 10-12 minutes to leave the stomach. NOTE: After you have taken the emulsified Cod liver oil and milk drink you cannot drink any water or any other drink for 1 hour as stated above.

Cold water is not recommended. Cold water will influence the digestive parts in the stomach. For this reason it is not recommended to drink cold water before the emulsified Cod liver oil drink. The cooling effect will affect the digestive process of the emulsified Cod liver oil and milk.

Other water containing drinks, such as coffee, tea and other drinks takes more time to digest and leave the stomach due to the various ingredients of the drink which need to be digested so for all other drinks than room tempered or warm water calculate with the same digestive period as for food, which is 4 hours, to be on the safe side.

The reason for the food, snacks, medicine and drink restrictions, before and after you drink the emulsified Cod liver oil and milk drink is to make sure the emulsified Cod liver oil and milk drink is digested and processed correctly in the stomach, the duodenum with the gallbladder with its bile and the pancreas with its pancreatic enzymes and juices and the digestive pipe or small intestine pipe. Any interference in the digestive process of the emulsified Cod liver oil drink, from any other drink, food, snacks, medicine, capsules or any other item will influence the digestive processes and the transfer process of the Cod liver oil lipids into the correct transport channel into the circulating blood to reach the cells in the skin and body.

The guidelines to obtain a healthy level of the important lipids from the Cod liver oil into the cells of the skin and body sounds perhaps complex, but it is not as you will soon understand from the explanations as follows:

With the restriction on food, medicines, drinks and any other items, when is the best time to take the emulsified Cod liver oil and milk drink?

Personally I selected the early morning, for my emulsified Cod liver oil and milk drink. To give you an idea of what I do, I start my day, as I have been doing for many years with 1-2 glasses of room tempered or slightly warm water, first thing in the morning, before having anything else.

After my water drinks, I now wait the required period of 10-15 minutes, to ensure the water has left the stomach before I shake for 15 seconds and drink the room tempered and emulsified Cod liver oil and milk drink already prepared and stored in a screw top glass jar.

The milk and the Cod liver oil in the screw top glass jar I normally arrange in the evening before I go to bed. It is stored outside the fridge in the kitchen. It has room temperature and it is easy to shake and emulsify before I drink it, either in the morning or during the night, if I should be up during the night.

The waiting period of 10 to 15 minutes, after my water drinks is not wasted, if you decide to follow my procedure of taking the emulsified Cod liver oil and milk drink in the morning. I am sure you will also find something to do if you are in a rush. There is one note I should mention if you decide to brush your teeth during the 10-15 minutes waiting period. When you brush your teeth it is important not to swallow water during the brushing as the water will interfere in the digestion. If you should swallow water during the brushing before you take your emulsified Cod liver oil you have to fit it into the schedule so the water does not interrupt the 10-15 minutes waiting period between water and the emulsified Cod liver oil drink. This is the time for the water to leave the stomach. If you should swallow some water during the 1 hour waiting period after you have taken the emulsified Cod liver oil it will interfere in the digestion and you have lost the healing power of the Cod liver oil for that day. Next day do better!

Basically all you have to do is to reorganize a few things of your morning routines and it should work out fine, even if you are in a rush. Planning is all what is required. I have even heard that some people get up earlier in the morning to fit in the emulsified Cod liver oil drink. After all you do not need to do it every day for life. Why not reserve 6-8 months of your life to insure against future health problems due to lack of the important Omega 3 and vitamin D?

When you have filled up your cells in the skin and body with the important lipids you will only need to take it once a week to replenish the healthy lipids.

Another very good time to take the emulsified Cod liver oil and milk drink, for some people, might be during the night, in case you have the habit to go to the toilet during the night. If you should follow this timing of taking the emulsified Cod liver oil remember the required 4 hours from your last meal, snacks or medicine. In this case it is also recommended to prepare the Cod liver oil and milk drink in the evening before going to bed. Leave the screw top glass jar in the kitchen or the bathroom during the night so it is ready to shake it before you drink it.

After taking the emulsified Cod liver oil drink you can go back to bed and sleep for the required 1 hour waiting time or more.

Coffee or tea as the first drink in the morning is not recommended if you want to take the emulsified Cod liver oil drink in the morning. Both the coffee and the tea will involve the digestion differently than water due to the herbal or bean ingredients in the drinks. So if you decide that you need your coffee or tea in the early morning you have to select another time for your emulsified Cod liver oil and milk drink.

You may take the emulsified Cod liver oil and milk drink just before bedtime if you feel this is a more convenient time. In this case you also have to remember the 4 hours after your last meal, snack or medicine.

If you feel that you need more than water, or Cod liver oil first thing in the morning, raw fruit, except bananas, will do fine as most raw and ripe fruit with high water content digest normally within 30-45 minutes. One exception to this rule is bananas, which have low water content. For this reason a ripe banana will require approximately 1 hour or more for complete digestion, all depending on the ripeness of the fruit.

As stated above, room tempered or warm water needs 10-12 minutes on its own and most raw fruit, except bananas, pass normally through the stomach in 30-45 minutes on its own. The rapid digestion or break down of the fresh fruit is due to their built in food enzymes which help to digest or break down the fruit very fast in the stomach.

Should you decide to have water and fresh fruits in the morning, before you take your emulsified Cod liver oil drink, remember to drink the room tempered or warm water a few minutes before the fruit. Water first will not interfere in the digestion. When you eat the fruit and drink the water together or drink the water after the fruit the digestion will be slightly delayed.

If you should wonder why I drink slightly warm water instead of room tempered water it is something I discovered in one old health book. According to the writer the warm water after it has been transferred into the blood and is moving towards the kidneys for processing it will help the kidneys to clean out toxins in the kidneys. It sounds logic, I thought, as you can easily see it is a very big difference in the result if you try to clean a plate of fat or grease with cold water, room tempered or warm water.

With this type of fruit breakfast get into the habit to drink your one or more glasses of room tempered or warm water first thing in the morning as soon as you get up and then wait a few minutes before you take the fresh ripe watery fruit. Altogether you will need a minimum of 45 minutes for this healthy alkaline fresh watery fruit breakfast, before you can take the emulsified Cod liver oil drink.

An alkaline fresh fruit breakfast high in water on its own will also over time support you health. Your blood is in need of the minerals, trace minerals and other ingredients of the fresh alkaline fruit and vegetables to stay in the healthy alkaline range. The high water content and fibre of the fresh fruit will help to clean out the walls in your intestine and colon pipe.

The morning time, part of the body's natural elimination cycle, is the best time to start with fresh watery and alkaline fruits.

My breakfast for the last 15 years or more has been mostly a very light fresh fruit and vegetable breakfast, after my water, with an apple or some other fresh fruit if available and some carrots, all organic if possible. Due to my emulsified Cod liver oil drink, I have now changed my breakfast routines. Now for breakfast, I drink my room tempered or slightly warm water first thing in the morning and then I start to prepare my apple and carrot breakfast or something similar during the 10-15 minutes waiting period, before I shake and drink my emulsified Cod liver oil and milk drink. My apple and carrot sticks I take 1 hour or more after my emulsified Cod liver oil and milk drink.

Should you want to reduce weight, the fresh watery fruit for the morning breakfast is a good way to start the weight reduction. I lost 22 kg and several numbers in shirt and jacket size in 1995, by changing my breakfast to fresh watery fruit in the morning plus following the food combining method of eating for the other meals during the day. The food combining method of eating is originally a very old method of eating to obtain a correct digestion of the food with the separation of protein and carbohydrates in each meal with lots of salads and vegetables. With this method of eating I can eat anything without thinking about calories and without having a weight problem. I still have the same weight I had back in 1995 and wear the same size of shirts I did wear when I was around 25 years of age.

Another good thing with this way of eating is the energy you get! Sorry for being carried away into a complete different subject, but as it is still related to health, why not.

Should the morning, evening or night time as mentioned above not be a good time for the emulsified Cod liver oil and milk drink for whatever reason you might find time to take the emulsified Cod liver oil and milk drink before your mid day or lunch meal. Again you need to remember Guideline 1 and 2 i.e. take the emulsified Cod liver oil and milk drink on an empty stomach with no food, snacks, medicines or any other items for 1 hour afterwards.

Should you become thirsty in the morning you are allowed to drink room tempered or warm water up to 10-15 minutes before you take your emulsified Cod liver oil and milk drink. Room tempered water will also normally stop the first hunger from developing.

Remember also that you should not eat or drink anything for one hour after taking the emulsified Cod liver oil and milk drink, so if you plan to take the drink before your lunch meal you need to plan accordingly.

What do I do if I am travelling and would like to take my emulsified Cod liver oil and milk drink?

Due to the travel restrictions with liquids on planes these days you need to plan accordingly, but as a table spoon of cod liver oil a day is such a small quantity of liquid it should be possible to fill it into one very small sealable plastic bag or small container. Whole milk is available almost everywhere. If you do not bring the screw top glass jar for the emulsifying process buy instead the milk in a small plastic bottle and use the small plastic bottle for the emulsification process.

Without following these simple food and drink guidelines to help the digestive system to digest and emulsify the Cod liver oil correctly, your cells in the skin, hair and body will not receive a healthy level of the important lipids Omega 3 and vitamin A & D and other lipids and ingredients from the Cod liver oil to start a healing process at the cellular level.

The progress with the emulsified Cod liver oil can be checked by inspecting the moistness of the skin on the hands and legs during the first two to three months and compare the results with the notes of the document.

How long do I need to take the emulsified Cod liver oil?

To heal the dry cells in the skin and body it is recommended to take the emulsified Cod liver oil drink with the lipids Omega 3 and vitamin A & D every day for a period of approximately 6 months. When your skin and body are very dry it can even take some more time. It sounds long, but when your cells in your skin and body are dry the only method to refill the missing and healthy lipids for the cells is to utilize the body's own distribution system to the cells via the blood circulation. The refill of lipids at the cellular level is a time consuming process which cannot be rushed. Gradually, day by day the cells throughout the body will be filled with up with the healthy lipids starting with the skin.

When you feel your skin has become soft and moist and has improved to the level you consider satisfactory and the other warning signals for lack of lipids are covered, you should not stop suddenly to take the emulsified Cod liver oil drink. Instead it is recommended to reduce it gradually to every second day for a period of one to two months. Thereafter it should be sufficient to take the drink only once a week. This weekly emulsified Cod liver oil drink will normally give you a healthy level of Omega 3 and vitamin D and the other lipids in the skin and body. This weekly supplementation is more or less the same as the very old recommendation of having a good fat fish meal once a week.

The condition of your skin or the colour of your ear wax will give you an indication or warning if you should need to increase the weekly emulsified Cod liver oil supplementation.

When will I start to see or feel a difference in my skin?

The time it will take for you to feel and see a difference in your skin, will depend on the dryness of the cells in your skin when you started. From my own experience and other peoples experience you need to take the emulsified Cod liver oil daily, for a period of approximately 1-3 months before you can expect to see and feel the first real difference in your skin. The skin on the hands and legs seems to be the first areas of improvements and then gradually improvements will move to the skin in the face and other parts of the body. From my own experience, with very dry skin, I noticed visible differences on my hands and legs after only approx. 1 ½ month, but it took approximately 2-3 months before I could feel and see a difference in my face.

Remember, if it should take longer than 6 months to obtain soft and moist skin your dryness is more than skin deep. All the trillion of cells in the body are at more or less the same dryness level as the cells in the skin due to the lack of the important lipids. The dryness you see and feel in the skin is the warning signal that something is wrong with the lipid level in all the cells in the body. Rough skin under the sole on your feet or on your heel is another area to watch for sign of dryness or cracked skin. This dryness is nothing else than a warning signal of lack of the important lipids at the cellular level, throughout the body. With dryness at the cellular level inflammation and other problems develop over time.

Another part of the body to check for lipids is the ears. Your ears should produce soft yellow ear wax if your body is not too dry. With age the earwax can turn dark or disappear altogether, which is another warning signal that the internal machinery is running out of lipids and is getting far too dry, with the risk of associated health problems. A correction of lack of yellow earwax can take 8-12 months.

Should you have crusty stuff in the corners of your eyes in the morning, you will notice the crust will disappear altogether after you have refilled your lipid stores.

When you have completed the emulsified Cod liver oil supplementation your skin should feel soft and moist, without dryness and without being oily. If you had oily skin or part of your skin was oily, the emulsified Cod liver oil treatment should over time help to remove the oily skin patches.

When you have reached the stage of soft moist skin the small wrinkles which come with dry skin might also slowly soften and disappear, if they are not too deep. The cells in the skin will gradually expand with the lipids from inside, the natural way.

The Cod liver oil, with the lipids Omega 3 and vitamin A & D and the other lipids and ingredients, contains some of the best nutrients nature can provide to help to maintain your skins natural youthful appearance.

Over time you might also start to feel improvements inside your body which should be much more important for your health than the improvement you will see and feel on your skin.

Something to consider when you have special health conditions.

Cod liver oil is a natural product which has been used by people to improve health for hundreds of years. The same somehow applies to whole milk even if the health aspect of whole milk was changed with the introduction of the pasteurization process during the early years of the 1900. With this long use as a medicine or food there should not be much to consider if you take this health drink based on Cod liver oil and milk.

There are different suppliers of Cod liver oil in the market, but in Norway the oldest and largest supplier of Cod liver oil is Peter Moller, established in 1854.

The Norwegian manufacturer, Peter Moller, does not state any real medical considerations on their bottles of "Tran" which is the typical Norwegian name for Cod liver oil in Norway. The only consideration they give, which is stated on the label of the bottle, is to reduce the daily dose of Cod liver oil for babies. According to them babies can be given 2, 5 ml Cod liver oil which is the equivalent to one teaspoon a day with a gradual increase to the normal adult dose of 5 ml which is equivalent to one normal tablespoon a day when the baby reach the age of 6 months. They inform on the bottle that it is not recommended to increase the daily serving size.

The same applies to the "Carlson Norwegian" Cod liver oil, which is also supplied by Peter Moller. They also recommend a daily serving size of 5 ml. They have not indicated any difference in serving size between babies or adults on the label on the bottle.

In Norway, the bottle of "Moller's Tran" is still considered as a medicine. The bottle or the label on the bottle has the statement "Medisintran" included which means it is considered as a medicine based on Cod liver oil. This is more or less the same medical declaration used by Dr. de Jongh back in 1850 when he introduced his Norwegian Cod liver oil as medicine to the public in Europe and the USA.

There are other manufacturers of Cod liver oil, but according to the medical and chemical testing performed by Dr. de Jongh in the 1850's, Cod liver oil should come from the cod fish living in the cold arctic waters. The cod fish living in these cold waters would have the diet required to give the Cod liver oil its medical healing power, to classify it as a medicine.

Dr. de Jongh, based on many years of research, concluded that the best Cod liver oil came from the cod fish from the cold arctic waters of Norway. Dr. de Jongh started to sell his Norwegian Cod liver oil as medicine in the 1850's and it was a tested and guaranteed product. The same applies to the Peter Moller or Moller's Tran or Cod liver oil and the "Carlsons Norwegian" Cod liver oil today.

As with all thing new, and Cod liver oil might be new for some people, even if this natural food and medicine product has been used for a very long time by many people, it is always recommended to start out with a test period to determine what can be the correct serving size.

In this respect some people might have difficult to digest fats or oils in food due to a troublesome gall bladder or if the gall bladder is removed. In such cases it is recommended to test out the correct amount of Cod liver oil in the milk to use. Perhaps the recommended dose of Cod liver for new born babies can be used as a guideline or perhaps a tea spoon on every second day can be used. Only an individual testing over some period of time will give the correct serving size if you should have digestive problem with fats and oils, but even with a troublesome or missing gallbladder your cells in your body will be in need of the essential fatty acid Omega 3 with DHA and EPA and the oil soluble vitamin A and D, which all are a natural part of the Cod liver oil. Should you decide to try the Cod liver oil emulsified in fresh orange juice, with all the fruit pulp removed, the same recommendations of testing will apply as not all people can handle fresh orange juice without some reactions in the stomach or body. In such a case the whole milk is recommended.

Omega 3 and vitamin A & D metabolism, simplified by an engineer.

When we analyse the research on healthy oils and their metabolism inside the cells in humans, two doctors stand out. Both doctors after their research, considered their discovery so important for health they decided to make their research available to the public in the 1940s-50s.

One doctor is Abraham White from the USA, who studied illnesses of the metabolism and lipid metabolism. With his study he tried to find a method to bring the essential fatty acid Omega 3 and the oil soluble vitamin A & D into the cell to prevent and heal illnesses associated with the lack of these important lipids at the cellular level. The other doctor is Johanna Budwig from Germany who studied fats and the healing of illnesses at the cellular level caused by a faulty metabolism of fat.

Their research or discoveries are not related in any way, but their method of changing the different type of healthy unsaturated oils with an emulsification or mixing process with another ingredient to reach the cells in the body via the blood circulation and the capillaries to achieve the targeted healing at the cellular level are almost identical.

Both doctors used natural food as their medicine, which had been the tradition in the medical field for thousands of years. Dr. A. White used Cod liver oil emulsified or mixed in whole milk and

Dr. J. Budwig used flax seed oil or linseed oil emulsified or mixed in low fat quark or cottage cheese.

What did they do?
Let us start briefly with the lady doctor.

Dr. Johanna Budwig/ 1908-2003, Germany, was a biochemist with a Ph.D. degree in medical education and an expert on fats and oils in the German fat industry. She studied fats and health most of her life and during her studies she discovered that chemically processed fats and margarine would over time cause malfunctions at the cellular level with the development of serious illnesses. With this discovery she decided to study healthy oils and their metabolism with the aim to find a healthy oil which could be made to circulate in the blood into the small capillaries to start a healing process at the cellular level. Dr. J. Budwig discovered after more than 20 years of research that flax seed oil, emulsified with a sulphur rich protein would be able to enter the blood circulation and flow with the blood into the cells to detoxify and bring oxygen at the cellular level. For the sulphur rich protein she decided to use low fat quark which is the German equivalent to the English cottage cheese.

With this simple food related medicine based on flax seed oil or linseed oil emulsified or mixed with quark and supported by a special diet including coconut oil as fat, she cured for many years patients in Germany with cancer, cardiovascular illnesses, arthritis and other illnesses

Dr. Abraham White/ 1908-1980, USA, was a biochemist and assistant professor at a university in the USA with a Ph.D. degree in Physiological Chemistry with strong interest in research and education. With the discovery of the oil soluble vitamin A and D and the essential fatty acid Omega 3 in the early 1900, the doctors were of the opinion that without a sufficient level of these essential lipids at the cellular level various illnesses could develop. Dry skin was seen as a warning signal for lack of these important lipids with a dry body. With these new discoveries Dr.

A. White decided to study lipid metabolism with marine oils or Cod liver oil, known to be rich in Omega 3 and vitamin A & D. He had previously researched the metabolism of different amino acids so he was well prepared for the research on lipids with marine oil or Cod liver oil.

Dr. A. White discovered with his study that water or any other watery drink during the meal, with food rich in the lipids Omega 3 and vitamin A & D, had a large influence on the correct digestion and transport of the important lipids. The water prevented the lipids to reach the cells in the skin and body in a sufficient healthy level to prevent dry skin and body. With his research he discovered water or any watery drink interfered in the digestion of the lipids Omega 3 and the oil soluble vitamin A and D present in marine oil or food rich in these lipids. The water or any other watery drink prevented a natural emulsification or break down process of the lipids during the digestion resulting in an incorrect absorption and transport of the important lipids in the body.

The second main reason for dry skin and body, he discovered, was the lack of an additional main emulsification process during the digestion for the lipids Omega 3 and vitamin A & D in the marine oil or food rich in these lipids. He discovered it was necessary to include an additional emulsification process in the meal to obtain more of the healthy lipids into the cells in the skin. Homemade soup with the meal, which had been a tradition in the families for generations if not thousands of years, would function as the additional emulsification process for the important lipids. He discovered room tempered or warm whole milk would do the same. At that time, few families in the city, had time to make homemade soups and many used canned or tinned soups instead, if any soup at all.

Doctors at that time used the condition of the skin to evaluate the health condition of the body. For them the skin was considered as the barometer for the health condition of the body. The development of the first paper chromatography for the analysis of the lipids in the blood did not come until after 1950, according to Dr. J. Budwig, who was one of the first doctors to try it out with her research on the fat metabolism.

Dr. Johanna Budwig is world famous for her research on fats and their related illnesses, and with her discovery of the emulsified flax seed oil or linseed oil and quark or cottage cheese to heal what is very often termed incurable illnesses. Dr. A. White did not manage to bring his important discovery with a healthy level of the lipids Omega 3 and vitamin A & D to prevent dry skin and body to heal or prevent illnesses associated with the lack of these lipids to the front pages of the news papers as Dr. J. Budwig managed with her cures of incurable illnesses. Had it not been for another person in the USA, Mr. Dale Alexander, in search for a cure for arthritis for his mother, Dr. A. White's research on lipid metabolism with his important discovery on how to obtain a healthy level of Omega 3 and vitamin D and the other lipids would most likely been forgotten. Not because Dr. A. White failed in his research, but because he did not manage to fight for his controversial, but important discovery, like Dr. J. Budwig.

For this reason the public in need of his research, for the health of their skin and body did not receive Dr. A. White's important information on Omega 3 and vitamin D through the news. His controversial study of lipid metabolism was instead presented as a chapter in a medical book with the title "Diseases of Metabolism". Hardly a book most people would buy, with the exception of Mr. Dale Alexander and probably a few others. Mr. Dale Alexander, who was not a doctor, was in search of medical information to cure his mother's arthritis which no doctor had managed to cure. He studied the work of Dr. A. White on lipid metabolism and understood how to use it to heal his mother's arthritis. In 1952 Mr. D. Alexander published his own book on a cure for arthritis and became famous in the USA. In an interview with Mr. D. Alexander, published in 1993, after more than 40 years of success with his book on arthritis and thousands of appearances in radio and TV, Mr. Dale Alexander informed the journalist who questioned him where he had got the information on the water's influence on the lipids and the use of Cod liver oil and milk. Mr.

Dale Alexander informed that his information on water and lipids and Cod liver oil and milk came from a study published by Dr. A. White as "Lipid metabolism" in a medical book "Diseases of Metabolism", as highlighted earlier. My small work contribution to the Omega 3 and vitamin D secrets have been to test it out and try to understand how water and lipids together can affect and have affected our health so negatively for such a long period of time. In the beginning I did not believe in the emulsified Cod liver oil study so I had to test it out. After I noticed it worked other people tested it out too. I am glad I did as it improved my health and I am sure it will improve your health too, if you test it out.

As far as I understand the lipids Omega 3 and vitamin D have secret powers. Medical science will continue to discover more and more of these secret powers. These secret powers kept our ancestors running for thousands of years. Hopefully I will be able to share my health discovery, with a healthy level of Omega 3 and vitamin D, to prevent or reduce a number of illnesses with a large group of people.

Should you try to study the old work of Dr. A. White, as Mr D. Alexander did, you will discover the doctor modified his study in his more recent publications on the lipid metabolism to let his study fit the opinion of the established medical view regarding the transport of the healthy lipids in the body. You will however discover that he never gave up completely the discovery of the second transport channel for the lipids into the blood circulation, via the lymphatic system. With this chapter I have tried to understand his discovery of the important second transport channel via the lymphatic system to bring a healthy level of the important lipids to all the cells in the skin and body. Please do understand that my guess work is only an engineer's view on a rather complex system which is a part of your body's immune system.

The emulsified Cod liver oil and milk method will still reach the cells in your skin and body at a healthy level, if you test it out, even if you do not follow my guess work.

Until there will be new research on healthy oils and their metabolism, we can use the available information for the correct use of marine oil or Cod liver oil and flax seed oil or linseed oil to guide us to obtain various natural healing effects in the body.

Dr. J. Budwig discovered that flax seed oil needed to be mixed or emulsified in a sulphur rich protein such as low fat quark or cottage cheese to reach the circulating blood and the capillaries feeding all the cells.

The capillaries are the name of the fine or invisible blood vessels, smaller than the human hair, where only one blood cell at a time will pass through. The capillaries reach each cell in the body and bring oxygen, nutrients and lipids from the circulating blood to the cells.

Dr. J. Budwig used the method with emulsified flax seed oil and low fat quark to heal cancer, arthritis, heart problems and other difficult illnesses for years, but had problems to get her treatment method accepted by the German medical establishment as her cure was considered a food and not a medicine. Dr. J. Budwig was taken several times to court in Germany by her medical colleagues, trying to stop her promoting her food medicine, but as her cure worked and she had well documented proof of healing with many patients she was never charged by the courts. Dr. J. Budwig never managed to get her emulsified flax seed oil treatment approved as a medicine by the medical authority in Germany. These days some doctors in Germany seem to have started to offer the Budwig treatment.

Dr. A. White discovered, like Dr. J. Budwig, the unsaturated marine oil or Cod liver oil rich in the lipids Omega 3 and vitamin D and other lipids needed an ingredient to emulsify the lipids to make the lipids more absorbable in the blood circulation feeding oxygen, lipids and other nutrients to the cells via the capillaries.

To obtain a natural emulsification process of the lipids in the digestive process he discovered the lipids in the marine oil or food had to be digested without water or any other watery drink, which he defined as an oil-free beverage, during the entire period of digestion. Without this separation between water and food rich in the important lipids, during the meal, very little or only between 5 % to 20 % of the available lipids in the marine oil or food rich in these lipids would reach the cells in the skin and body depending on the temperature of the watery drink consumed with the food.

Cold water or cold drinks with food, which had become popular at the time of his research, reduced the transport of the healthy lipids Omega 3 and vitamin D into the cells of the skin and body to almost zero or 5 % of the available lipids in the marine oil or food.

When water or any other watery drink was separated from the food and consumed at least 10 minutes or more before the food, so the water would have time to leave the stomach before the arrival of the food in the stomach, and up to 3 hours after the food to complete the digestion of the food, he discovered the water would not interfere in the digestion and the natural emulsification process of the lipids. With this separation of water and food a much higher percentage of the lipids in the marine oil or food with up to 50 % of the available lipids would reach the cells in the skin and body.

To obtain a much higher absorption level of the lipids Omega 3 and vitamin D into the cells of the skin and body from marine oil or food rich in these lipids Dr. A White discovered in addition to the separation of the water and food, the food rich in lipids had to receive an additional emulsification process to emulsify more of the lipids in the food. He discovered homemade soups and room tempered whole milk or warm whole milk would emulsify the marine oil or food rich in these lipids as both the soup and the whole milk, separately, would increase the lipid penetration into the cells of the skin and body with up to 95 % of the available lipids in the marine oil or food rich in lipids.

The doctor discovered also that canned or tinned soup products did not have the ability to emulsify the oil or lipids and could not be used to emulsify the lipids. He discovered the soups had to be homemade with fresh products to give the required emulsifying process to the available lipids to obtain a high additional level of the important lipids into the cells of the skin.

Fresh orange juice, where all the pulp or fibre of the fresh juice had been removed would also act as an emulsifying liquid for the lipids Omega 3 and vitamin A & D and give a high percentage of the lipids into the cells of the skin and body, but the fresh orange juice has to be free of any pulp.

With his discovery on how to obtain a healthy level of the lipids Omega 3 and vitamin A & D and other lipids present in marine oil or Cod liver oil, which I have tried to describe, I hope you will now understand why many of us get dry skin and body after years of good food or marine oil supplements considered to be rich in these important lipids.

Our habit of drinking cold watery drinks or even room tempered or warm watery drinks during or after our meals during the 3 hour digestive process is the main reasons why we do not manage to get a healthy level of the important lipids from the food or supplements rich in these lipids. The water or the other watery drinks prevent a natural emulsification process of the lipids during the digestive process which is required for the lipids to enter the correct transport channel into the body to reach all the cells in need of the lipids throughout the body. Instead the important lipids end up in the wrong transport channel and the wrong organ in the body where the important lipids cannot do much to help to prevent dry skin and body and the associated illnesses.

Previous generations avoided to a large extent the problems associated with the lack of the healthy lipids due to their diet with homemade soups and their habit of separating water and food in most of their meals. They had also a more natural exposure to the sun. They were used to drink their water when they were thirsty when they came home to eat and rest. With this habit of drinking water before the food which had to be heated, they had to wait. The food consisted most likely of a thick soup or stew several times a week. With this natural habit they separated water and food. After the food a rest after a long day with work was probably normal. With this habit of drinking water before the food and a rest after the food they obtain a long natural separation between water and food, most of the time. This natural habit of drinking water, eating and resting enabled them to obtain a healthy level of Omega 3 and vitamin D from food rich in these lipids, most of the days, without thinking about it.

As long as we continue our habit to drink water or any other watery drink with the food it would not help us to use the homemade soup or stew to try to increase the absorption rate of the important lipids. The water or any other watery drink taken during the digestive period of the food will prevent a natural emulsification process of the lipids. This emulsification process is required for the correct absorption of the lipids into the correct transport channel feeding the cells in the skin and body.

From his discovery of the correct metabolism of the important lipids it seems Dr. A. White understood, contrary to normal medical understanding at the time, the circulating blood had more than one supply channel to obtain the important lipids Omega 3 and vitamin A & D, but 2 different supply channels from the same source or digestive pipe or intestine pipe. Both the supply or transport channels extract their molecular lipid parts from the same intestine pipe, after the digestion, but the function or operation of the transport channels are completely different.

When Dr. A. White started his research he knew from the people with dry skin that very little of the important lipids Omega 3 and vitamin A & D would reach the cells in the skin via the normal transport channel via the circulating blood passing through the kidneys and the liver when water or any other watery drink was consumed together with the food. Perhaps he was aware of previous research made by other doctors and people long before his research pointing out that water had to be consumed before the food and approximately 3 hours after the food for the digestion to obtain maximum nutrients from the food.

From his research it seems the digestive process in the stomach and the first part of the intestine pipe can be compared to a chemical process. Much like a chemical process in a factory where the various digestive parts, juices and enzymes will all act together, and like any chemical process when the incoming ingredients are changed and mixed the outgoing end product from the chemical digestive process will change. In such a chemical process different molecular end products will be produced and this is exactly what is happening in our digestive process, when we add or remove water from the chemical digestive process.

By applying the chemical digestive process idea to our complex digestive process we can consider the digestive pipe or intestine pipe to be the receiving station for the output molecular end products from the first chemical digestive process. At this receiving station different molecular end products arrive from the digestive process ready to be processed into the next transport channel or channels moving or extracting the molecular end products from the intestine pipe to the inside of the body.

Before we start to look at the chemical digestive process idea of the digestion let us first look briefly at the available infrastructure in the intestine pipe. This infrastructure will be involved in the processing or extraction of the different molecular end products arriving in the intestine pipe after the digestive process.

The internal wall in digestive pipe or the intestine pipe is covered by billions of small tap-off valves named villus, designed to absorb the molecular end products entering the intestine pipe. Inside each villus there are 2 different types of villi, which is another smaller type of tap-off valve. Each villi tap-off valve is connected with a small tube to their respective main transport channel or vein located or embedded directly on outside wall of the intestine pipe. All the two different types of villi tap-off valves are connected in parallel to their respective transport channel or vein. One transport channel or vein is leading into the portal blood flowing towards the liver and the second transport channel or vein is leading into the lymphatic fluid flowing towards the Thoracic duct.

One type of the villi tap-off valve is programmed to operate only for the correct emulsified and molecular lipid end products Omega 3 and vitamin A & D and other lipids, with no fresh water molecules or any other fresh water molecules present. The other type of the villi tap-off valve does not have this water limitation program to absorb molecular end products. They can operate on almost any molecular end product passing by in the intestine pipe inclusive all the lipid molecular end products with water or any other watery molecules. For this reason this type of villi is considered to be the main villi tap-off valve for the molecular end products for the cells in the body.

Both the villie tap-off valves with their respective transport channels transport their molecular end products to the same circulating blood, feeding all the cells, after cleaning and processing.

The main villi tap-off valves which are programmed to absorb almost any molecular end products with water and without water from the intestine pipe are designed to transporting the molecular end products into the transport channel with the portal blood leading the molecular end products to the kidneys and the liver for cleaning and processing. This main transport channel with its large cleaning facility in the kidneys and the liver is designed to handle many types of different molecular end products. The liver will however finally decide what nutrients of molecular end products to store, to dispose as waste or to pass on into the new blood, before the blood is refreshed with oxygen from the lungs, and pumped into a new blood circulation and distributed again via the capillaries into all the cells.

The second villi tap-off valves which are programmed to open and operate only with the correct emulsified and molecular lipids Omega 3 and vitamin A & D and the other healthy lipids without any water is designed to transport the emulsified and molecular lipid end products into its own transport channel. This transport channel will lead the emulsified and molecular lipid end products into the lymphatic system with the lymph with the lymphatic nodes, Cisternae chyli and the Thoracic duct for cleaning and processing. The Thoracic duct is designed to pass the lymph with the reassembled and emulsified and molecular lipid end products directly into the new circulating blood feeding the capillaries leading to the cells. The tap-off villi valves for this transport channel leading into the lymphatic system and the circulating blood is designed to open without water. In this no water condition it is designed to absorb the correct emulsified and molecular lipid end products. Due to our relative new habit of drinking water or any other watery drink during the digestion of the food these types of villi tap-off valves will remain closed for a very large percentage of the population. For previous generations, who had the habit of drinking their water when thirsty and normally before their food and long after their food, these villi tap-off valves would be open when people consumed their food. With our relative new habit of drinking water or any other watery drink with our food containing the important lipids these very important villi tap-off valves leading into the lymphatic transport channel will remain closed most of the time.

To recap the actual discovery of Dr. A. White:
Food with water would give only 5 to 20 % of the molecular lipid end product of Omega 3 and vitamin D and the other lipids to the cells in the skin, depending on the temperature of the water, compared to approximately 50 % without any watery drink. Homemade soup or room tempered or warm whole milk, without water, would increase the lipid penetration into the cells from 50 % up to 95 % of the available lipids.

With his discovery of the different levels of the important lipids in the skin with water or no water and homemade soups or milk the following 3 meal situations can be used as a simple explanation for the 2 different transport channels for the movement of the lipids in the body. Both transport channels will lead the important lipids into the circulating blood feeding the capillaries and all the cells, but only one transport channel is able to bring a healthy level of Omega 3 and vitamin D into the cells in the skin and body. The transport channel via the lymphatic system is the new correct transport channel for the important lipids Omega 3 and the oil soluble vitamin D plus the other oil soluble vitamins. Unfortunately this very important transport channel designed to protect our health is closed when we drink water or any other watery drink, with our food. For our ancestors this was not a problem, as they had a different habit of drinking water as already explained.

Meal situation 1. A meal with food rich in Omega 3 and vitamin A & D with water or any other watery drink present during the 3 hours digestive process:

In this meal situation, which is a very normal meal situation for most people these days, the type of villi tap-off valves programmed to open and absorb for almost all the molecular end products, with water or without water, inclusive the healthy lipids, would open and absorb all the molecular end products reduced to a molecular size fitting the villi tap-off valves. These villi tap-off valves would open and absorb the lipid molecular end products every time there would be water or any other watery drink with the food preventing a natural and correct emulsification process during the digestive process. The villi tap-off valves will lead the molecular end products into the transport channel for the portal blood with the kidneys and the liver. The kidneys and the liver will filter and sort the different molecular end products. As soon as the liver receives the molecular end products of the lipids Omega 3 and vitamin A & D and other lipids it will either store the important lipids, send some of the lipids into the blood to be used for the new blood circulation or start to use the lipids as energy for heating. Depending on the temperature of the incoming molecular end products the liver is handling it will use more of the important lipids or less of the lipids for its own heating process and protection to keep a stable temperature in the body. Lots of cold molecular end products arriving with cold drinks would require more heat to be generated by the liver to keep the temperature and only up to 5 % of the available lipid molecular end products received would be released by the liver into the new blood circulation.

Meal situation 2. A meal with the same type of food, but with no entry of water or any other watery drink during the 3 hours digestive process:

In this meal situation, the digestive process would manage to emulsify a lot of the lipids Omega 3 and vitamin A & D and other lipids in the food, but not all of the lipids in the food would be emulsified. When all these molecular lipid end products enter into the intestine pipe, with no fresh water molecules, the villi tap-off valves for the lymphatic system, programmed to open only for the correct emulsified lipids, will now open and manage to extract all the correct emulsified and molecular lipid end products Omega 3 and vitamin A & D and other lipids. The rest of the molecular lipid end products Omega 3 and vitamin A & D and other lipids which did not receive a full and correct emulsification process during the digestive process will pass into the villi tap-off valves connected to the transport channel or vein leading into the portal blood where the kidneys and the liver will clean and process the lipids. Again very little of the lipid molecular end products entering into the main villi tap-off valves leading to the kidneys and the liver will be released into the new blood circulation. This time, without water, when a good portion of the important lipids in the food received a correct emulsification process during the digestion and entered the second transport channel, via the lymphatic system, designed to operate only for the correct emulsified lipids, much more of the important lipids reach the cells in the skin and body. With this method of eating with no water or any other watery drink during the digestion Dr. A White estimated that 50 % of the available lipids Omega 3 and vitamin

A & D and other lipids in the marine oil or food rich in the lipids would reach the cells of the skin and body.

Meal situation 3. A meal with the same type of food, and again with no water or any other watery drink during the 3 hours digestive process, but with a homemade soup or room tempered or warm whole milk added during the digestive process:

In this meal situation, the digestive process would manage to emulsify correctly almost all the lipids Omega 3 and vitamin A & D and other lipids in the marine oil or food. When this almost 100 % correct emulsified and molecular lipid end product mixture enter the intestine pipe after the digestion, with no water molecules or any other fresh water molecules present, the villi tap-off valves for the lymphatic transport channel would open and this time manage to extract almost all the correctly emulsified molecular lipid end products Omega 3 and vitamin A & D and the other lipids. The small rest amount of the lipid molecular end products with an incomplete emulsification process after the digestion would pass into the main villi tap-off valves for the portal blood to be processed as explained earlier. With this method of eating with homemade soup or warm or room tempered milk and no water or any other watery drink during the digestion Dr. A. White estimated 95 % of the important lipids available in the marine oil or food rich in the lipids would reach the cells in the skin and body.

As soon as we start to combine marine oil or food rich in lipids with water or any other watery drink during the meal, the villi tap-off valves designed to handle only the correct emulsified and molecular lipid end products Omega 3 and vitamin A & D and the other lipids will be closed or blocked. With the villi-tap-off valves leading into the transport channel via the lymphatic system closed the lipid molecular end products Omega 3 and vitamin A & D and the other lipids will instead have to pass through the main villi tap-off valves leading into the portal blood with the kidneys and the liver. The entry of the important lipids Omega 3 and vitamin A & D and the other lipids into this main transport channel, considered to be the "normal" transport channel into the cells in the body, will as we know, result in a low distribution level of the healthy lipids into the blood circulation feeding the cells of the skin and body.

The low distribution of the important lipids into the cells will result in dry cells in the skin and body with the risk of associated illnesses.

The transport channel via the lymphatic system for the important lipids was the transport channel Dr. A. White discovered, with his study of marine oil or Cod liver oil in the 1940s, but it seems he failed to fight for the discovery of this mostly passive transport channel for the important lipids Omega 3 and vitamin A & D. Perhaps he understood the difficulty he would face to try to change the medical opinion that the human body had more than one transport channel for the lipids Omega 3 and vitamin A & D and the other lipids into the circulating blood and the cells? Perhaps he also understood that the days with food medicine, which worked, were over? Most likely he encountered the same problem as Dr. J. Budwig encountered with her food medicine in Germany. For whatever reason his discovery was not really understood or accepted by doctors in need of his discovery for their patients.

The transport channel via the lymphatic system into the blood circulation is probably the transport channel discovered by some other doctors much earlier when they noticed the separation of the food and water improved the digestion with better health. The cells in the body received more healthy lipids!

The final process of the lipid metabolism will be reached as soon as the molecular end products of the lipids Omega 3 and vitamin A & D and the other lipids reach the cells via the blood circulation, but there is no need for you to evaluate or consider the many complex processes and functions which are part of the lipid metabolism inside the cells.

Instead you can focus on the end results of the correct lipid metabolism in your skin. Since the discovery of the lipids Omega 3 and vitamin A & D in the early years of the 1900 doctors have known that lack the important lipids in the cells will cause dry skin and body. They knew also that this dryness at the cellular level carried risk for certain illnesses. When you get soft moist skin you know the cells in the skin have received a healthy level of the important lipids via the blood circulation. The same applies to all the other trillions of cells in your body. The soft moist skin you obtain is the proof of the correct lipid metabolism with the healthy lipids, as Dr. A. White discovered with his study.

The evaluation of the skin condition was the method used by the doctors in the old days to judge the health condition of a person. According to them, your skin is the barometer of your health. It mirrors the condition of the body at the cellular level.

One important point to consider is that the study of the Cod liver oil metabolism with Omega 3 and vitamin A & D or food rich in these lipids was performed before the blood tests for the lipids were invented.

The doctor had to focus his research on the lipid metabolism with marine oil or Cod liver oil on the end product of his research, the softness of the cells in the skin, all the time. At that time he could not measure the actual flow of the molecular lipid end products in the lymph, the blood or the intestine after the digestion. Instead he established a method of measuring the softness or lipid penetration of the Omega 3 and vitamin A & D and other lipids into the cells of the skin. This gave him a tool to evaluate the correct lipid metabolism of the healthy lipids in marine oil or Cod liver oil or food rich in these important lipids at the cellular level. Perhaps this was his advantage compared to do the research today, based on a blood test for the lipids?

By now, I hope you understand the doctor discovered something very important for the cells of your skin and body and your health.

His research work is somehow backed by the new research work performed by two universities, one in Europe and one the USA, these days. It seems these two universities independent of each other are concluding that we need 10 times or even more of the important oil soluble vitamin D than the present daily recommendations. It seems we need this high protective and preventive level to protect us for some of the most serious illnesses we are facing today.

Perhaps this was the level of vitamin D previous generations received with their outdoor work and natural habit of drinking water, when thirsty, before their food and long after their food which most likely consisted of thick homemade soups or stews, most of the days?

These days, the "Vitamin D Council", a private organization, involved in the study of illnesses related to the lack of the oil soluble vitamin D has concluded we are reaching or have reached a worldwide vitamin D deficiency of epidemic proportions with more than one billion people at risk for associated illnesses.

The problem with the lack of the important essential fatty acid Omega 3 and oil soluble vitamin D is much more complex today than 50 years ago. The problem now is not only related to our relative new habit of drinking water or any other watery drink with food or lack of homemade soups and sun exposure, but it is also related to our modern diet. A diet based on industrial farming. An industrial farming which produce food with low level of the natural Omega 3 and vitamin D due to grain feed or other unnatural type of feed to increase weight and reduce cost. Instead we risk getting much higher level of Omega 6 and a synthetic form of vitamin D with form D2 which is being added to some important food sources instead of the natural and important vitamin D form D3.

The discovery made by Dr. A. White in the 1940s with the correct absorption, transport and lipid metabolism of the lipids in the Cod liver oil is easy to test. You follow the supplementation method with the emulsified Cod liver oil and milk which is based on meal situation 3. With this method approximately 95 % of the available lipids in the Cod liver oil will be distributed to the cells in your skin and body. You will see it first with your skin. Your skin will become moist and soft.

When you can feel soft and moist skin after approximately 1-3 months, depending on your dryness when you started, you know that the lipids are entering the cells in the body as the skin is the first organ which will benefit from a healthy level of Omega 3 and vitamin D and the other lipids.

Do not take my word for it, but for your own health sake take the time to test it out. Within a few months you will have the proof of the lipid penetration into the cells of the skin and body. You will have soft and most skin!

Later on you might also notice other healthy changes in your body as these important lipids are involved in many more cellular processes in all the 100 trillion cells than what is known today.

Another good thing with the supplementation method with emulsified Cod liver oil is the high level of Omega 3 in the Cod liver oil will help to counteract a possible high level of the lipid Omega 6 in the body obtain from vegetable oils, snacks and food high in Omega 6 oils. At the same time you will also receive a healthy level of the natural oil soluble vitamin D together with a good level of the oil soluble vitamin A.

Old medical studies indicate the oil soluble vitamin D needs the oil soluble vitamin A to function properly. In Cod liver oil both the lipids exist naturally together.

We need water, but we should know when to drink the water.

Your body is approximately 70% water. The percentages between solid matter and water varies for men and women, fat or skinny and old or young, but on the average the water content is between 60%-75 %. The level of water will also depend on which source you use to obtain the water data. Irrespective of what water level is correct, the body is mostly water. The body uses a kind of emulsified water mixed with trace minerals or salts. Your digestive system starting with the saliva when you chew your food until the waste products leaves the body uses lots of emulsified water. This sea of internal water needs to be topped up on a daily basis with new pure water of good quality.

Drink water when you are thirsty have been and still is the normal recommendation, but is this a good recommendation?

What did our ancestors do?

They drank their water when they were thirsty, most of the time. For them water was not available as tap water or in bottles. With their problem to carry water we can assume the first thing they would do when they came home to eat and rest would be to drink water to stop their thirst before doing anything else. Their food most likely consisted of a thick soup or stew, which had to be heated. After the food they would most likely rest or sleep after a long day of work. With this natural habit of drinking water, when thirsty, before the food they would also separate water and food correctly most of the time, without knowing it.

Without obtaining sufficient pure water, we would be dehydrated.

Dehydration would slowly affect all ongoing processes in the body, is the statement we normally hear or read. Few doctors are able to give you a good explanation on how much water your body would need, except the advice to drink water when you feel thirsty or up to 2-3 litres a day.

There seems to be no real long term medical study on how much water you need to drink to maintain good health over time, but there are different medical studies on water and health to improve the digestion to obtain more nourishment from your food.

From the research performed by Dr. A. White on lipid metabolism with marine oil or Cod liver oil to obtain the important lipids Omega 3 and vitamin A & D to correct dry skin and body we know the important lipids in the food will not reach all the cells in the skin and body when we drink water or any other watery drink with our food rich in lipids. There are also other older studies in the USA and Europe on water, food and health and even more recent studies on the same subject which all have come to more or less the same conclusion. Water and food have to be separated in a meal to give good digestion. With a good digestion your body will use less digestive enzymes to digest or break down the food and you will obtain more nutrients from the food to improve health.

Dr. F. Batmanghelidj/ 1931-2004, was an Iranian doctor, with a UK medical education. He started his study on water in Iran during the Iranian revolution when they had a shortage of medication for digestive ulcers. After the Iranian revolution he moved to the USA where he had the opportunity to continue his medical research on water and health for more than 20 years. He discovered what some other doctors had discovered before him, you need to separate water and food to obtain a good digestion.

According to the research made by Dr. F. Batmanghelidj and Dr. A. White and other doctors before them who studied water, food and health, you should drink your water before your food with no water for a period of 3 hours after the food. According to the Iranian doctor the water takes approximately 30 minutes to pass through the stomach into the intestine pipe where it will be processed, absorbed and emulsified or mixed into the blood. After this process the water will be ready to support digestion with digestive juices. It seems that Dr. A. White discovered with his study of the lipids that the first part of the water`s journey into the body and blood could be reduced to 10-15 minutes. The separation between the water and food these doctors discovered with their research will ensure the body uses less enzymes and energy to digest the food and at the same time receives more nutrients from the food.

In this respect, I would like to mention again the mother and uncle of my German wife, living in Hamburg, who celebrated their 87th and 93rd birthday in 2010. They followed this habit of drinking water with the separation of water and food in their meals when they were young. Their parents had learned this habit of separating water and food from their parents to protect their health. Other families in the same area followed the same habit of separating water and food.

Dehydration seems to be a normal situation these days, according to Dr. F. Batmanghelidj. The reason is the consumption of the many types of soft drinks, sports drinks, tea, coffee and all the other watery drinks. These drinks have to a large extent replaced pure water for many people. According to the doctor these drinks do not count as water, even if they contain water. The digestive system and the kidneys will use equal amount of water and some more water from the body to try to digest the drinks and flush out the toxins in the drinks. The extra water needed for the digestion and the detoxification processes, will be extracted from the water inside the cells and the blood, which will cause even more dehydration and problems.

According to the Iranian doctor every doctor knows water is important. Our body is a marine environment, but very little medical study has been made on the water metabolism and dehydration and the early signs or symptom of dehydration. Dehydration is a disturbance of the water metabolism where the body is suffering from a chronic water shortage. A chronic water shortage will over time lead to digestive problems and dry body. Both symptoms can lead to many serious illnesses.

Thirst is the first warning signal the water level in the blood and the cells of the body are far too low, according to Dr. F. Batmanghelidj. According to him you need, when you consume a normal diet of food where the food will also contain some water, learn to drink water correctly. You need approximately 6 glasses of water during the day to avoid being dehydrated.

The morning time is the best time of the day to start to fill up your water level in the body. The recommendation is to drink one or two glasses of room tempered water in the early morning as soon as you wake up. The other glasses of room tempered water should be consumed 10-30 minutes before your meal and 3 hours after the meal with the last glass of water to be taken before you go to bed assuming that you do not eat too late in the evening to obtain the 3 hour separation between food and water.

Water plays a very active role in the many chemical processes in the body inclusive the digestive system with the stomach and pancreas. The stomach and the pancreas need water to function properly for its production of the pancreatic digestive enzymes and digestive juices.

Water is also the main source of energy and water help to reduce stress in the body.

From the research performed by Dr. A. White we know water with food rich in the lipids Omega 3 and vitamin A & D will prevent the correct digestion and transport of the lipids to the cells in the skin and body. This situation will over time cause dry cells in the skin and body, with the risk for associated illnesses.

Lack of water in the body with dehydration as a result is another serious problem. Should you have reached the stage with certain small digestive discomforts, these discomforts might be caused by dehydration.

Dehydration together with lack of trace minerals from food can result in low stomach acid. With low stomach acid the production of the digestive enzyme Pepsin responsible for the digestion or break down of the protein part of the food in the stomach will be affected. With a too weak or low Pepsin level, due to a too low stomach acid, the protein part of the food will not be digested or broken down to the required molecular size in the stomach. The undigested protein part of the food is transferred from the stomach into to the next digestive process, in the duodenum with the pancreas and the gallbladder. The duodenum is the first short part of the long digestive pipe or intestine pipe connected between the stomach and the anus. In the duodenum both the pancreas and the gall bladder are active to digest and break down all the molecular sized food particles arriving from the stomach to smaller molecular particles before the small molecular particles move into the intestine pipe to be absorbed into the body.

When the pancreas receives the partly undigested protein food particles or molecules from the stomach the pancreas will have to work overtime to produce strong pancreatic enzymes and digestive juices to try to complete the break down process of the partly undigested protein food molecules arriving from the stomach with each meal. This additional pancreatic work load with the partly undigested protein part of the food will continue for every meal. Slowly over the months and years the pancreas will be overloaded. When this happens there is a high risk that the pancreas will fail to break down the protein part of the food to the correct molecular size required for the transfer process into the blood and body. Without a correction, with the correct natural ingredients like water, minerals and trace minerals, the situation with the overloaded pancreas will only become worse over time. More and more of the undigested protein food particles will enter the intestine pipe together with the digested protein food particles. Some of the undigested protein food particles will unfortunately manage to be absorbed into the blood. Now your immune system will have to work overtime to detoxify or eliminate the incoming undigested protein food particles in the blood seen as toxins.

An overload of the immune system can easily lead to more serious malfunctions of the immune system with the development of serious illnesses, over time.

From the increased sale of the medication antacids, which is used to calm down the stomach by changing the stomach acid strength, there is an indication that these small digestive problems, caused mainly by a lack of water and trace minerals, is increasing in many countries.

If you have digestive problems small or large you have reached a stage of dehydration, according to Dr. F. Batmanghelidj. According to him it seems that most people are dehydrated even without knowing it due to the large consumption of all the many new watery drinks where the water is not really the water the body needs to stay healthy.

How do you check if you are hydrated or dehydrated?

According to Dr. F. Batmanghelidj, the colour of the urine for a fully hydrated person should be almost clear to light yellow in colour. Dark coloured urine, without taking any vitamins or medicine, which can turn the urine to bright yellow or another colour shade, can be a good indication of dehydration.

Dehydration will also increase the acidity in the blood and body.

Acid accumulation in the blood and body over time will change the normal alkaline pH level of the blood into an acid pH level. Acid blood is the cause of almost all illness according to two doctors who researched health in the early years of the 1900 in the USA and Germany, such as Dr. William Howard Hay/1866-1940 and Dr. Gunther Enderlein/1872-1968. According to Dr. W. H. Hay acid accumulation in the blood and body is a self-inflicted situation, caused by a diet with food and drinks high in acids. When the blood and body reach an unhealthy and acid pH level illness has a chance to develop.

Our situation with acid food and drinks has not improved. On the contrary we have these days a very high consumption of processed and refined food and drinks, high in acids. A diet with too much carbohydrate or starchy food and protein food is one of the reasons for the development of acid blood and body. Another main reason is the high consumption of canned, bottled, and carton juices and other acid drinks, including the espressos and cappuccinos. They all give an acid reaction in the blood and body.

Pure water with a pH value of 7 is considered neutral on the pH scale. When you drink sufficient good water the water will prevent dehydration. The water will assist to bring about a less acid blood and body. The water after the absorption into the blood will also help to flush out toxins.

The pH scale or the "potential Hydrogen" scale is a logarithmic scale used to measure acid and alkaline solutions. On this scale 7 is neutral and everything below 7 is acid with 0 being the strongest acid. Everything above 7 is alkaline with 14 being the strongest alkaline solution. The pH scale can also be seen as a thermometer with 7 being the middle point of the thermometer. The bottom part can represent the acids and the upper part of the thermometer can represent the alkaline solutions. The end of the acid scale would be 0 and the end of the alkaline scale would be 14.

A diet high in alkaline food rich in minerals such as fresh fruit, berries, salads and vegetables will help to balance the intake of acid food and drinks. The alkaline food and drinks will move the pointer on the scale closer to a pH value of 7. Too much of the acid food and drinks such as bread, rice, meat, fish, cheese, yoghurt, milk, canned, carton and bottled juices and other drinks as well as coffee, tea etc will move the pointer into the acid range with a pH value below 7.

A healthy person has a blood pH value of approximately 7, 35, which is considered slightly alkaline. An acid body will normally have a blood pH value below 7 which is acid on the pH scale. To stay healthy your blood and body need to stay in the alkaline pH range. When we are born the blood is normally slightly alkaline with a normal pH level.

Our bodies to function properly are in need of the correct pH balance in the blood with a slightly alkaline level. There are thousands of ongoing processes in the body and they all depend on metabolic enzymes for their proper functions. Without a healthy alkaline pH level the performance of the metabolic enzymes will be affected and many important cellular processes in the blood and body will slow down. To protect itself the body will always try to find a way to compensate for too much acidity. To do this the blood or the blood cells will extract from the bones the minerals which give the fastest correction of the acidity such as calcium and magnesium and other minerals. Over time, if this is not compensated with alkaline food rich in minerals, this can lead to Osteoporosis.

The blood of a person has to be restored to a slightly alkaline pH level before a natural healing at the cellular level can take place, according to Dr. Gunther Enderlein.

When we consume lots of food and drinks high in acids the blood moves gradually to the acid side of the pH scale unless we are able to compensate for the build up of the acidity in the blood with pure water and alkaline food high in minerals and trace minerals. There are also other more modern reasons for the acid build up in the blood and body such as air pollution via the lungs and toxic pollution via the skin. The skin, being the largest organ receives a lot of toxins these days with the extensive use of hair shampoo, deodorants, cosmetics, skin lotions, creams and all the other add on skin layers containing toxic ingredients, including most sun creams or sprays.

To reduce or eliminate the build up of acidity in the blood and body you need to drink more pure water, instead of acid drinks, to avoid dehydration and to help the body to detoxify. You need also to eat more fresh alkaline food high in organic minerals, trace minerals and enzymes.

Fresh fruit, berries and vegetables, from good mineral rich soil should normally supply the trace minerals required to correct the acidity in the blood if you drink sufficient water. Pure water and mineral rich alkaline food with limited intake of good acid food has kept our ancestors walking and running for thousands of years. Unfortunate most soil these days due to the heavy agriculture food production with chemical fertilizers do not produce fruit, salads and vegetables rich in all the important minerals and trace minerals needed by the blood to stay alkaline.

Two important sources of organic minerals and trace minerals, not much used by many people are dry vegetables from the sea and unrefined sea salt from unpolluted sea areas. Today the sea is the richest source of the many important trace minerals or salts. The minerals have been washed into the sea from the soil and the mountains over millions of years. Regarding the use of dry sea vegetables to obtain the important trace minerals from the sea we can learn a lot from the Japanese people.

If your urine should turn out dark in colour, without the use of vitamins and medication, the body is dehydrated. The recommendation by Dr. F. Batmanghelidj, is not to rush to drink water, but instead organize your water drinking gradually according to the correct use of water. Start by drinking water

30 minutes before the meal and try to drink no water for up to 3 hours after the meal. The reason for this slow start is to give a dehydrated body time to adjust to the water. According to the doctor, if you are dehydrated, you need also to check that the kidneys are in good working condition and able to handle the filtration of the additional new water. To do this he recommends you to try to judge the amount of water entering is more or less equal to the amount of water leaving the body.

You should also try to remember your body is not designed to drink all these new acid drinks with all kinds of questionable refined sugar and chemical ingredients. Some of these acid drinks are more like a full meal and require a proper digestion like a full meal before they can be absorbed into the blood and body. This is an added burden on the pancreas with the additional production of digestive enzymes and juices. After the digestion of the drink with the absorption of all the molecular parts of the drink into the blood, the kidneys and the liver will try to clean out as much as possible of the toxic waste from the drink. Over time there will however be a gradual accumulation of various toxins in these organs, which will have an impact on their future performance.

Room tempered pure water on the other hand requires no involvement of the pancreas or the gall bladder and very little cleaning work by the kidneys and the liver. The blood and the cells in the skin and body in need of the water will love it.

Some of the necessary water, to avoid dehydration, can also be supplied from a diet with fresh raw fruit, berries, salad and vegetables high in water, preferably from areas with mineral rich soil. A diet with 70% mostly raw alkaline fruit, berries, salads and vegetables high in water and 30 % solid or cooked food will help to bring good water, enzymes, minerals and trace minerals into the blood to help the blood stay in the healthy alkaline pH range.

With the old habit of drinking water, before the food, which our ancestors used most of the time, for thousands of years, the water will not interfere in the digestion of the food. Instead more of the important lipids and trace minerals available in the food will reach the cells to support health.

Your stomach and body is not designed for cold drinks. The invention of the fridge is a relative new invention. According to the doctor who studied the lipid metabolism with marine oil, he discovered cold drinks will affect your digestion in such a way that hardly any of the healthy lipids in the food will reach the cells in your skin and body to support good health.

I know it can be difficult to break out of the existing habit of drinking water or any other watery drink with food, in the beginning. Try to get into the habit to drink your water 10 minutes or more before the food. Finish the drinks at least 10 minutes before the food. With water before the food you should not be thirsty so the second requirement with a waiting period of 3 hours after the food should also over time, be relatively easy to control for most meals, as it is only a habit. If you eat at restaurants regularly try to get into the habit to order your water or any other watery drinks immediately upon arrival before you start to study the menu. Finish the drinks 10 minutes before the food. Forget the waiter who wants to sell you drinks. It is part of his job. Take charge!

Should you reach a situation where you feel your body would benefit from some extra help to correct internal health issues consider the separation between water and food in your meals. With this habit of drinking water your body will use less enzymes and energy to digest the food. Your digestive system with the pancreas will function more correctly without having to use too much of the important metabolic enzymes to support the digestive processes and all the cells in your body will receive more of the healthy nutrients from the food. With more nutrients and the correct use of water the cells will be given a chance to detoxify and heal themselves over time.

The Iranian doctor used natural sea salt, preferably unrefined sea salt in his water cure. The unrefined sea salt with the water brings approximately 70 important trace minerals into the blood which will help to make the blood less acid.

The body is designed to heal itself, but the body needs to receive the correct lipids, water, trace minerals, enzymes and other nutrients.

Whenever possible when you are having a good meal rich in lipids, try to follow what your ancestors did for thousands of years. Include a homemade soup with your meal and follow the correct habit of drinking water or any other watery drink. The homemade soup will almost double the absorption rate of the important lipids into your cells in your skin and body, from 50% to 95%, as long as you do not include a watery drink in the meal, according to study of Dr. A. White.

The cells need the important lipids, but they also need the water, minerals, trace minerals and other nutrients.

Dr. F. Batmanghelidj used his water cure for his patients in the USA for more than 20 years to heal many illnesses. His water cure seems to be mostly based on nothing else than tap water with natural sea salt of a good quality. Good natural unrefined sea salt is rich in the important trace minerals. With the correct water cure and sea salt he claimed to have cured successfully illnesses for his patients related to digestive problems with ulcers, migraine, allergies, asthma and breathing problems, blood pressure, angina pain, low back pain, rheumatoid arthritis pain, depression, stress, other body pains and other illnesses.

Water with unrefined sea salt as medicine!

Think about it. How did he manage to be allowed to practice medicine with water and sea salt?

He researched water metabolism with the many functions of water in the body and presented his research papers to the medical authority in the USA. With his research he tried to have water classified or listed as medicine. It seems the medical authority could not prove him wrong, but they never approved water as medicine. He practised and used his water cure for many illnesses for many years and he never lost his medical practice! His Water cure is well documented with his books, with medical case stories. The books covering his water cures are available on his website watercure.com or from amazon.com.

I have recently started to follow the correct habit of drinking water or any other watery drinks with most of my main meals and I can feel something is changing to the better in my complex digestive system and body.

Remember also from the study performed by Dr. A. White that water and cold water or any other cold watery drink with food affects the digestion of the important lipids Omega 3 and vitamin D. The water and especially the cold water with your food will prevent almost all of the important lipids Omega 3 and the oil soluble vitamin D in the food to reach and benefit the cells in your skin and body. Water and lipids do not emulsify or mix!

Your body needs these important lipids for many functions. Your body can only obtain the lipids from food and the food has to be rich in lipids, but you have to give the body a chance to obtain it correctly. A too low level of Omega 3 and vitamin D at the cellular level carries certain health risk.

You might already have different insurances to cover risks for your car, residence, medical or other issues. Consider a healthy level of Omega 3 and vitamin D as your best health insurance. The good think with this health insurance is that you can check if the lipid insurance is working. You feel and see it with your new soft most skin.

Note: The habit of drinking water correctly is not a requirement to improve your dry skin, hair or body with Omega 3 and vitamin A & D and the other lipids if you follow the emulsified Cod liver oil and milk method, but it can help you with other health issues.

How do I start to improve my skin and body?

For you to obtain soft and moist skin the natural way with a healthy level of the lipids Omega 3 and vitamin D and the other oil soluble vitamins you have to follow the supplementation method discovered by the doctor who studied lipid metabolism with marine oil or Cod liver oil in the 1940s. The good thing with this method of supplying the missing lipids to the cells the natural way from the inside via the blood circulation is that all the cells in your body will receive the missing lipids. You will also be able to monitor the progress with the cellular healing with your skin.

To get started you need to buy the first bottle of Cod liver oil. When you buy the Cod liver oil, make sure the Cod liver oil is high quality with guaranteed values of Omega 3, DHA, EPA, Vitamin A, D and E. Normally these values of a good quality Cod liver oil are printed on the label of the bottle. There are other suppliers in the market, than the listed suppliers, but it is recommended to check their product and values and compare with the listed suppliers under the chapter, **"What type of marine oil to use as supplement, fish or Cod liver oil?"** and **"What type of Cod liver oil to use"**.

The Cod liver oil described comes normally in a 250ml bottle which is equivalent to 8, 4 ounces. The bottle should last approximately 50 days for an adult, based on a daily consumption of a full table spoon per day or 5 ml. Babies and children up to the age of

6 months need less and for them according to the Norwegian supplier of Cod liver oil, one tea spoon a day is sufficient.

It is recommended to buy more than one bottle of Cod liver oil when you start to avoid running out of supply.

The chapter or page, **"How do you obtain Omega 3 and vitamin D from Cod liver oil"** will give you a short overview of the correct supplementation method with Cod liver oil.

You will also need to buy a few small screw top glass jars to be used for the emulsification process. For more details regarding the selection of the correct sized screw top glass jars and how to use them, read the chapter **"How do you emulsify Cod liver oil"**.

To select the best time to drink the emulsified Cod liver oil, read the chapter **"When is the best time to take the emulsified Cod liver oil"**.

That's it.

The rest of the document or book you can read as and when you have the time to read it as this skin and body healing with the lipids Omega 3 and vitamin D and the other lipids will take more time than 14 days or 3 weeks. The complete healing process to fill up all the trillions of cells in the body lacking the important lipids takes at least 6 months, if not longer. The healing period will depend on the dryness of your cells in the skin and body when you start. During this waiting period to reach a healthy level of the important lipids in all your cells in your body you will be able to monitor your healing progress with your skin. First you will notice soft and moist skin and then gradually the lipids will fill up the cells deep inside the body. This deep cellular penetration of the healthy lipids might also over time, depending on your body's cellular dryness, introduce other more important positive changes in your body.

Consider the healing process with the important lipids Omega 3 and vitamin D and the other lipids as an insurance against future health problems. Your body will love you for it and already after 1-3 months, you should be able to see and feel the first real difference in your skin.

Reflections.

Illnesses related to the lack of the essential fatty acids Omega 3 with DHA and EPA and the oil soluble vitamin D are many and seems these days to increase. According to some doctors they might soon become a new health problem of unknown dimensions.

Previous generations had also certain health problems, but they did not have the same health problems related to dry skin and body due to lack of Omega 3 and vitamin D as we have today.

The lipid metabolism with marine oil or Cod liver oil and other healthy oils were studied extensively after the discovery of the oil soluble vitamin A and D and the essential fatty acid Omega 3 in the 1940s by doctors with the aim to bring the important lipids Omega 3 and vitamin A & D into the cells to avoid dry skin and body and the associated illnesses. After the Nobel Prize in Medicine was awarded in 1931 to Dr. Otto Warburg for his discovery of the transport and metabolism of oxygen in the cells different studies were also undertaken by doctors with the aim to bring oxygen into the cells to cure cancer.

One doctor in biochemistry in the USA who studied illnesses of the metabolism and lipid metabolism with marine oil or Cod liver oil to bring Omega 3 and vitamin A & D into the cells discovered water or any other watery drink when consumed with food with lipids would interfere in the digestion of the lipids. The water or any watery drink would prevent a correct digestion, emulsification, absorption and transport of the lipids into the cells of the skin and body. His discovery of the correct emulsification, absorption and transport of the essential fatty acid Omega 3 and the oil soluble vitamins to avoid dry skin and body seems to have passed unnoticed or considered an unimportant discovery by the medical community at that time. Today with a rapid increase in illnesses caused mainly by a lack of these important lipids due to wrong absorption and transport of the lipids, his discovery should be much more valuable.

In the 1970's there were studies of the lipid Omega 3 with DHA and the EPA with the Inuit tribe in Greenland which gave increased knowledge of the importance of the essential fatty acids to prevent cardiovascular problems, but the study did not bring any information on how to obtain the important lipids apart from eating more fish or food rich in the lipids.

Since then books upon books are written about the need of Omega 3 with DHA and EPA and the oil soluble vitamin D to improve health, but there are no guidance on how to obtain the important lipids, with the exception of the old general recommendation to increase the consumption of fish or consume more meat, eggs or other food considered to be rich in the important lipids.

If we follow this old recommendation we still get dry skin and body due to lack of Omega 3 and vitamin D and the other lipids with the associated illnesses. This should be the best proof that we still do not know how to obtain these lipids, even with the best food or supplements.

One dental doctor, who travelled around the world for extended periods of time studying the health of primitive and isolated populations in the 1920s and 30s, noticed the health of these people started to decline for each generation as soon as they started to adopt more to our new Western diet with refined sugar, white flour, salt and canned food products.

Considering we have an apparent large increase in new illnesses caused by the lack of Omega 3 and vitamin D and the incorrect digestion of fats it seems strange there are no research which is focused on the food with lipids and fats and their metabolism which seems to be the root problem of most illnesses these days. After all we have been following the same refined diet and habits for a much longer period of time than the isolated populations being studied by the dental doctor back in the 1920s and 30s. Instead most medical research, since the 1950s to improve health, seems to be focused on the study of new chemical medicines to try to control the illnesses with the use of medicine for life.

Another way to look at illnesses, from an engineering point of view, would be to consider that a large percentage of the illnesses we are having today are caused by accidents in the stomach with a faulty digestion of certain lipids and fats resulting in millions of serious problems or accidents. In engineering, with accidents, we would instead of spending all our effort to try to find something to control the problems or accidents focus most of our effort to identify the source of the problem, to prevent similar accidents. Compare it to an aircraft accident with the extensive and costly research to identify the cause of the problem to prevent similar accidents in the future.

With our digestive accidents caused mostly by our change of habits with our relative new habit of drinking water or any other watery drink with our food with lipids and fat, we have got millions of accidents resulting in costly illnesses and death each year, but hardly anything is done by the authorities to prevent or reduce the number of accidents.

Instead a very high percentage of the income of any Government is going towards an ever increasing health cost. To correct this unhealthy situation it feels logic that research on food with lipid and fat metabolism to be initiated by one of the ministries with the help of the universities. By dividing such a study between different universities the research, should be able to give results within a relative short period of time.

The cost for such research, with the correct information to the population on how to avoid certain illnesses related to an incorrect digestion and metabolism of oils and fats, would in a relative short period of time be covered by a reduction of the ever increasing medical cost. Less illness in the population would also normally result in higher productivity by the workforce in the country.

As far as I understand, it took the Dr. Johanna Budwig more than 20 years of research to find the simple emulsification process for the flaxseed oil with the result that emulsified flax seed oil could enter the blood circulation to reach the cells to detoxify old fats, bring oxygen and heal at the cellular level at the same time. The research on the lipid metabolism with marine oil or Cod liver oil to obtain the lipids Omega 3 and vitamin D and the other lipids by Dr. Abraham White took also several years, but he discovered the influence on water in the digestion of the lipids. Water and lipids do not mix and he discovered the mixing would prevent the correct digestion, emulsification, absorption and transport of the lipids into the cells in the skin and body. The research on the water metabolism and health took also Dr. Fereydoon Batmanghelidj more than 20 years.

A new and combined research on the illnesses of the metabolism with the lipid and fat metabolism with water and without any watery drink, starting with the research, performed by the above mentioned scientists, should give valuable knowledge within a relative short period of time. At the same time the research might be able to uncover the real working of the "sleeping" second transport channel into the blood circulation via the lymphatic system and the Thoracic duct.

Bibliography and sources.

1. Flax oil as a true aid against arthritis, heart infarction, cancer and other diseases, by Dr. Johanna Budwig. ISBN-0-9695272-1-7.
2. The oil protein diet, cookbook, by Dr. Johanna Budwig. ISBN-0-9695272-2-5.
3. Your body's many cries for water, by F. Batmanghelidj. M.D. ISBN-0-9629942-3-5.
4. Diseases of Metabolism, edited by Dr. Garfield G. Duncan. M.D. The book has many contributors, inclusive Dr. Abraham White, Ph.D.
5. Diseases of Metabolism, Second Edition. Detailed Methods of Diagnosis and Treatment, edited by Garfield G. Duncan. M.D. The book has many contributors, inclusive Dr. Abraham White. Ph.D.
6. Principles of Biochemistry, General Aspects, by Dr. Emil L. Smith, Ph.D., Dr. Robert L.Hill, Ph.D., Dr. I. Robert Lehman, Ph.D., Dr. Robert J. Lefkkowitz, M.D., Dr. Philip Handler, Ph.D., Dr. Abraham White, Ph.D. ISBN-0-07-069762-0.
7. Essentials of Rubins Pathology, 5th edition, by Dr. Emanuel Rubin, MD. Howard M. Reisner. Ph.D. ISBN-13:978-0-7817-7324-0/ ISBN-10:0-7817-7324-5.
8. Why stomach acid is good for you, by Jonathan V.Wright. M.D. and Lane Lenard, Ph.D. ISBN-0-87131-931-4.
9. Nutrition and physical degeneration, by Weston A.Price, D.D.S. ISBN-0-916764-08-7.

10. Food combining for health, A new look at the Hay system, by Doris Grant & Jean Joice. ISBN-0-7225-0882-4.

11. Food combining for life, by Doris Grant, ISBN-0-7225-3165-6.

12. Arthritis and Common Sense, by Dale Alexander. ISBN-978-0-671-42791-7.

13. Dry skin and Common sense, by Dale Alexander. ISBN-911638-05-9.

14. Biographical Memoir, Abraham White, 1908-1980, National Academy of Science, Washington D.C. by Emil L. Smith.

15. The LAST CHANCE Health Report, Special Edition, 1993, University of Natural Healing/ Virginia—USA. How to permanently eliminate dry skin. Interview with Dale Alexander, by Sam Biser.

16. Chapter 3—Vitamin D: Production, Metabolism, and Mechanisms of Action, by Daniel D. Bikle, M.D., Ph.D.

17. Vitamin D Newsletters, by Dr. John Cannell, MD, Executive Director Vitamin D Council.

18. Doctor's House Call, by Dr. Al Sears, MD. August 16, 2007. The most powerful cancer fighter ever discovered is naturally occurring vitamin D.

19. Metabolism at a glance, by Dr. J.G. Salway. ISBN-0-632-03258-8.

20. Norsk olje gjennom tusen ar. Lofoten som global Tran produsent, by Ottar Schiotz.

21. Inflammation, by Dr. H. O. Trowbridge, Dr. R.C. Emling. ISBN-0-86715-310-5.

22. Dead doctors don't lie, by Dr. Joel D. Wallach & Dr. Ma Lan.ISBN-1-880692-40-6.

23. Out of the Mainstream and into the light, a workshop health document, issued Sept.25, 1993, by Dr. Joel D. Wallach.

24. Dr. Jensens guide to better bowel care, by Dr. Bernard Jensen.ISBN-0-89529-584-9.

25. Foods that heal, by Dr. Bernard Jensen. ISBN-0-89529-563-6.

26. Vibrant health from your kitchen, by Bernard Jensen, Ph.D. ISBN-0-932615-01-5.
27. Colon health, by Norman W. Walker, D.Sc. ISBN-0-89019-069-0.
28. Water can undermine your health, by Norman W. Walker, D.Sc.ISBN-0-89019-037-2.
29. Vibrant health, by Dr. N. W. Walker. ISBN-0-89019-035-6.
30. Become younger, by Dr. N. W. Walker, D.Sc. ISBN-0-89019-051-8.
31. The digestive system, by Margaret E. Smith, PhD. D.Sc. & Dion G. Morton. M.D. D.Sc. ISBN: 978 0 443 06245 2.
32. Enzyme Nutrition, by Dr. Edward Howell. ISBN-0-89529-221-1.
33. The Missing Ingredient, by Lee Euler. ISBN-978-1-60402-610-8.
34. Salt, your way to health, by Dr. David Brownstein. M.D. ISBN-978-0-9660882-4-3.
35. Iodine, the most misunderstood nutrient, by Dr. David Brownstein. M.D. ISBN-978-0-9660882-3-6.
36. Iodine, why you need it, why you cannot live without it, by David Brownstein. M.D.
37. Iodine, Note-Book of Materia-Medica-1867, Pharmacology and Therapeutics, with a supplement introduced into, the British Pharmacopia of 1867, page 133-134, by Dr. R.E. Scoresby-Jackson. M.D. Edinburgh.
38. Vitaminer og Mineraler, by Dr. Matti Tolonen. ISBN-82-7410-003-4.
39. Enzymes for digestive health and nutritional health, by Karen DeFelice. ISBN-0-9725918-6-9.
40. Fats that heal, Fats that kill, by Udo Erasmus. ISBN-0-920470-38-6.
41. We tell the story of Chemistry. Chemical Heritage Foundation, by Diane Wendt.
42. Key contributions to medicine. John Hughes Bennett Laboratory, Leukaemia research fund, The University of Edinburgh.

43. Essential cell biology, by Dr. B. Alberts, Dr. D. Bray, Dr.K. Hopkin, Dr. A. Johnson, Dr. J. Lewis, Dr.M. Raff, Dr.K. Roberts, Dr. P. Walter. ISBN-0-8153-3481-8.
44. Immunology, by Prof. Dr. I. Roitt, Prof. Dr. J. Brostoff, Dr. D. Male.
45. The liver cleansing diet, by Dr. Sandra Cabot. ISBN-0-646-27789-8.
46. Coconut Cures, by Bruce Fife, N.D. ISBN-0-941599-60-4.
47. The truth about coconut oil: Why it got a bad rep when it is actually good, by Dr. Joseph Mercula—email customer service. Sept 2003.
48. New look at coconut oil. The Weston Price Foundation for Wise Traditions, by Dr. Mary G. Enig, Ph.D.
49. A Cancer Therapy, Results of fifty cases, by Dr. Max Gerson, M.D. ISBN-0-9611526-2-1.
50. Healing, the Gerson way, by Charlotte Gerson. ISBN-978-0-9760186-2-9.
51. How to fight cancer & win, by William L. Fisher. Agora Health books.
52. O2XYGEN Therapies, by Ed McCabe. ISBN-0-9620527-0-1.
53. The Cure for all Diseases, by Dr. Hulda Regehr Clark, Ph.D., N.D. ISBN-1-890035-01-7.
54. Diet Wise, Let your body choose the food that is right for you, by Prof. Keith Scott-Mumby M.B., Ch.B., M.D., Ph.D. ISBN-13:978-0-9768617-1-3 & ISBN-10:0-9768617-1-2.
55. Take control of your health, by Dr. Joseph Mercola with Dr. Kendra Pearsall. ISBN: 978-0-9705574-1-4.
56. Fit for life, by Harvey and Marilyn Diamond. ISBN-0-553-17355-3
57. Why suffer?, by Ann Wigmore. ISBN-0-89529-286-6.
58. The metabolic typing diet, by William Wolcott and Trish Fahey. ISBN-0-7679-0564-4.
59. Eat right for your type, 4 blood types, 4 diets, by Dr. Peter J. D'Adamo. ISBN-0-399-14255-X.
60. Live right for your type, by Dr. Peter J.D' Adamo. ISBN-0-7181-4476-7.

61. Dr. Atkins Age-defying Diet revolution, by Dr. Robert Atkins. ISBN-0-09-182547-4.
62. The nature doctor, by Dr. H.C. A. Vogel ISBN-1-85158-274-6.
63. Nutritional Medicine, by Dr. Stephen Davies & Dr. Alan Stewart. ISBN-0-330-28833-4.
64. Surviving into the 21st Century-Planetary Healers manual, by Viktoras Kulvinskas. ISBN-0-933278-04-7.
65. Food for thought, your guide to healthy eating, by Vernon Coleman. ISBN-1-898947-97-X.
66. Surviving the toxic crisis, understanding, preventing and treating the root causes of chronic illness, by Dr. William R. Kellas. Ph.D and Dr. Andrea Sharon Dworking. N.D. ISBN-0-9636491-2-4 and ISBN-0-9636491-1-6.
67. The WDDTY guide to Good Digestion, by Lynne McTaggart. A WDDTY publication.
68. Natural Way to Health. Monthly health publication, by Dr. David Brownstein. 2008-2011.
69. The Douglass Report. Monthly health publication, by William Campbell Douglass II, M.D. 2000-2011.
70. The Blaylock Wellness report. Vitamin D's hidden role in your health, by Dr. R. L. Blaylock. M.D. Sept. 2008. Vol. 5, No. 9.
71. The Blaylock Wellness report. Omega 3, Nature's Miracle Panacea, by Dr. R.L. Blaylock.M.D. April 2005. Vol. 2, No.4.
72. To Your Health. Monthly health publication, by Dr. John A. McDougall. 2001-2006.
73. Health & Longevity. Monthly health publication, by Dr. Robert D. Willix Jr.1995-1999.
74. What doctors don't tell you (WDDTY), Monthly health publication.1999-2009.
75. Second Opinion Health Alert. Monthly health publication, by Dr. Robert J. Rowen. 2009-2011.
76. Doctor's House Call, Monthly and weekly Health Alerts, by Dr. Al Sears M.D. 2004-2011.
77. Guide to Good Health, The hidden danger of stomach-acid reducers, by Dr. Allan Spreen. M.D.

78. Health Science Institute, HSI. Monthly health publication. 2002-2010.
79. Nutrition & Healing. Monthly health publication, by Dr. Jonathan V. Wright. 2002-2011.
80. Fat may be the healthiest food you can eat. Health document, by Dr. David Eifrig. The Stansberry & Associates.
81. Financial Times, Monday, May 5, 1997. Advertising. Finding new ways, Hoechst.
82. The internet and the Wikipedia, the free encyclopaedia.